THE EXPRESSIVE LIVES OF ELDERS

MATERIAL
VERNACULARS

Jason Baird Jackson, *editor*

# THE EXPRESSIVE LIVES OF ELDERS

*Folklore, Art, and Aging*

Edited by Jon Kay

Indiana University Press, in cooperation with the

Mathers Museum of World Cultures, Indiana University

*This book is a publication of*

Indiana University Press
Office of Scholarly Publishing
Herman B Wells Library 350
1320 East 10th Street
Bloomington, Indiana 47405 USA

iupress.indiana.edu

A free digital edition of this book is available at IUScholarWorks:
http://hdl.handle.net/2022/22075

Manufactured in the United States of America

Cataloging information is available from the Library of Congress.

ISBN 978-0-253-03707-7 (hardback)
ISBN 978-0-253-03708-4 (paperback)
ISBN 978-0-253-03711-4 (ebook)

1 2 3 4 5    23 22 21 20 19 18

This edited volume is dedicated to the memory of

*Alan Jabbour:*

folklorist, fiddler, friend

# Contents

Acknowledgments                                                                                                          *ix*

Introduction:
Folklore and the Expressive Lives of Elders / Jon Kay                                                                     *1*

PART I. Observations on Folklore and Aging

1   Boot Lasts and Basket Lists:
    Joe Patrickus's Customized Art and Life / Lisa L. Higgins                                                            *27*

2   Aging with Grace and Power:
    A Puerto Rican Healer's Story / Selina Morales                                                                       *42*

3   Fieldworker in the Cane:
    A Puerto Rican Life History in Wood and Words /
    Julián Antonio Carrillo                                                                                              *55*

4   The Role of Traditional Arts in Identity Creation in the
    Lives of Elders / Patricia A. Atkinson                                                                               *80*

5   "I Don't Have Time to Be Bored":
    Creativity of a Senior Weaver / Yvonne R. Lockwood                                                                   *95*

6   Still Working: Performing Productivity through Gardening and
    Home Canning / Danille Elise Christensen                                                                            *106*

7   Quilts and Aging / Clare Luz and Marsha MacDowell                                                                   *138*

8   Curating Time's Body: Elders as Stewards of
    Historical Sensibility / Mary Hufford                                                                               *153*

PART II. Folklife and Creative Aging Programs

**9** Elderhood Arts / Kathleen Mundell     *175*

**10** Dancing Chairs and Mythic Trees: The Power of Folk Arts
in Creative Aging, Health, and Wellness / Troyd Geist     *186*

Index     *205*

# Acknowledgments

From the beginning of this book project, I wanted to enlist authors who could write from rich firsthand experiences. I thank the eleven contributing authors who generously penned their insights into their respective chapters to make *The Expressive Lives of Elders: Folklore, Art, and Aging* a readable and actionable collection of essays. This book, however, also benefited greatly from the perceptive suggestions of two engaged peer reviewers whom I thank for their contributions to the shaping of this book. I also thank Jason Baird Jackson, the Material Vernacular Series editor, for his thoughtful direction on this project.

Throughout various stages of this project, student workers helped with the formatting and compiling of the manuscripts. Thanks go to Dom Tartaglia, Micah Ling, Evangeline Mee, Katlin Suiter, Emily Hunsicker, and Donald Bradley for their work on this project.

Gary Dunham and his team at Indiana University Press made this project a reality. At the 2016 Annual Meeting of the American Folklore Society, Gary suggested an edited volume on folklore and aging. The next year, several of the volume's authors contributed papers to two panels on the topic for the 2017 annual meeting. After the conference, Janice Frisch and Kate Schramm at the press worked their magic, helping me stay on track and on time with this project. Their dedicated efforts and gentle reminders helped bring this collection into existence.

I am thankful for the scholars and elders whose words and influence informed these essays. From Barbara Myerhoff and Barbara Kirshenblatt-Gimblett to Alan Jabbour and Simon Bronner, several scholars have broadened and deepened our understanding of the expressive lives of older adults. The observations offered in this volume came from the contributors working with dozens of older adults who shared their lives, talents, and insights with us. While the names of the elders who helped shape this book are too numerous to list here, I would acknowledge Joseph F. Patrickus Jr. (1947–2018) for his contribution to this project as his life was drawing to an end. I am appreciative of him and the many unnamed older adults who collaborated with the authors of this volume.

THE EXPRESSIVE LIVES OF ELDERS

# Introduction

## *Folklore and the Expressive Lives of Elders*

### Jon Kay

From 1997 to 2004, I worked as the folklorist at the Stephen Foster Folk Culture Center in White Springs, Florida. This was my first long-term position as a public folklorist, which meant that I was based in a community for an extended period. As the folklorist for this state park, I coordinated craft demonstrations, produced public events, and hosted Elderhostel programs. Looking back on those years, it was then that I began thinking earnestly about the expressive lives of older adults: that is, how the stories, foods, crafts, games, music, and other forms of traditional knowledge that a person accumulates throughout their life become a valuable resource for them as they reach an advanced age. This is what this edited volume explores—the creative practices of older adults and how elders use these expressive forms in their daily lives.

While working at the Folk Culture Center, I witnessed how traditional arts not only supported older adults in later life but also helped many to thrive well into their eighties and nineties. Each fall, the center hosted a festival called Rural Folklife Days, a multiday celebration of local traditions. Most of the participants at the event were of retirement age; this group of elder quilters, blacksmiths, cane syrup makers, jelly canners, checkers players, musicians, and storytellers shared skills they learned in their youth with thousands of schoolchildren (fig. 0.1). While the event aimed to teach the students about local history and cultural practices, I quickly realized that the older artists got as much or perhaps more out of the event as the students. In addition to the small stipend the park paid the demonstrators for their participation in the event, each elder was rewarded with the opportunity to share their life stories and special skills with the young attendees. I recognized that these demonstrators were not like many older adults

*The Expressive Lives of Elders* (2018): 1–24, DOI: 10.2979/expressivelivesofelders.0.0.01

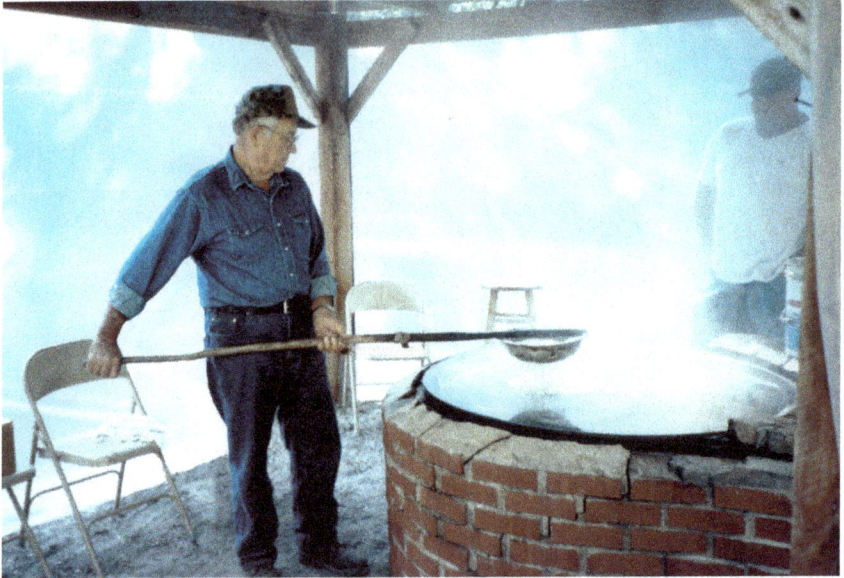

Fig. 0.1. Ivy Harris making cane syrup at Rural Folklife Days in White Springs, Florida, 2002. *Photograph by Jon Kay.*

in the United States, who suffer from isolation, boredom, and helplessness (Yale 2004). Instead, these elders were connected, engaged, and capable. I found the elders involved in this public program inspiring, and they contributed much to my understanding of life as a whole—not just the folklife they were hired to present. Programs such as Rural Folklife Days are not unique in the work of public folklorists in the United States. From the Smithsonian Folklife Festival on the National Mall to an African drumming workshop at a local library, folklorists work with older tradition bearers to help them share their personal experiences and talents with the public. However, folklorists seldom focus on how the programs and events they produce may work to improve the quality of life of the older participants.

Recently, I was hosting a limestone-carving program at a state park in Indiana, when out of the corner of my eye, I saw an older artist whom I had worked with a few years earlier. Glenn Hall's daughter had driven the ninety-three-year-old man to the event. "He made me bring him here to see you!" she explained. "Long time no see, Mr. Hall," I said to the retired farmer turned metal sculptor. "It was May the fifth 2012 at the Patoka Festival," he replied. His daughter stared at him and asked, "How did you remember that?" "Well, it was just about the best day of my life," he explained. The one-day festival at which Glenn had demon-

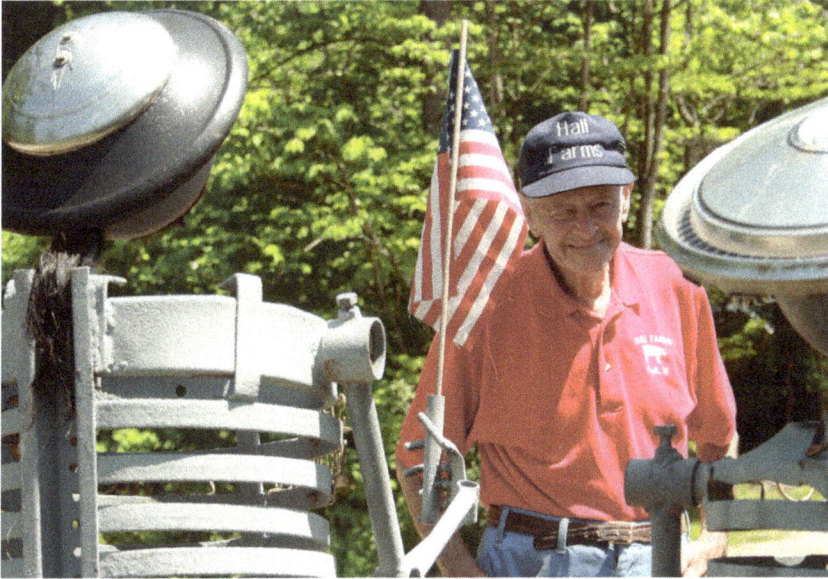

Fig. 0.2. Glenn Hall at Patoka State Park with his metal sculptures, 2012. *Courtesy of Traditional Arts Indiana.*

strated was just one of several arts programs that I helped produced that year (fig. 0.2). I had enjoyed watching Glenn interact with visitors at the festival but had given little thought to what his participation meant to him. As this book demonstrates, the projects and programs that folklorists facilitate benefit the lives of older adults. Currently, these culture programs are primarily designed to support community engagement and demonstrate the artistic excellence of an art form or artist, per National Endowment for the Arts guidelines. However, public folklore theories, methods, and models, I believe, can also be deployed to improve the lives of older adults.

For example, folklorists study the dynamic ways that stories, art, food, music, dance, play, and similar expressive forms help build and support our social lives. When Dan Ben-Amos (1972) redefined folklore as "artistic communication in small groups," he foregrounded both the communicative and social aspects of expressive forms. Similarly, Richard Bauman (1972, 33) encouraged folklorists to study "the social base of folklore in terms of the actual place of the lore in social relationships and its use in communicative interaction." My years of studying the social interactions of older adults has confirmed for me that jam sessions, quilting bees, bocce ball tournaments, writing clubs, and morning coffee klatches help elders constitute and maintain their social ties. Gerontologists now recog-

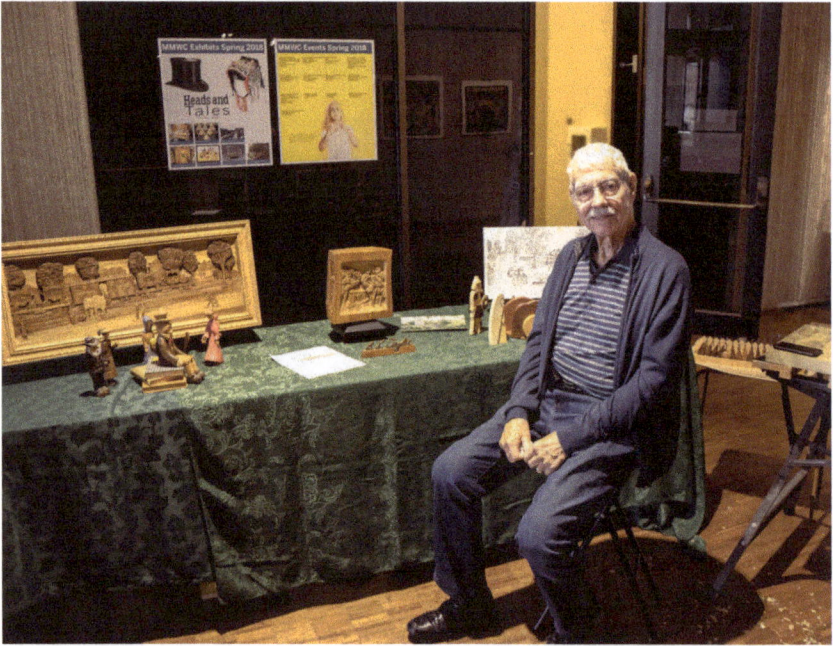

Fig. 0.3. Bob Taylor with his circus carving at the Mathers Museum of World Cultures at Indiana University, Bloomington, 2018. *Photograph by Jon Kay.*

nized that these small groups and social networks are essential for maintaining an elder's health and wellness in later life. A 2015 study reviewed data from more than three hundred thousand people over a seven-year period and found that individuals with good social relationships were more than twice as likely to continue to live than people with poor social relationships. This means that creating and maintaining social connections is comparable to quitting smoking as a predictor of living longer. In fact, isolation and loneliness seem to surpass obesity and a sedentary lifestyle as risk factors for mortality in later life (Holt-Sunstad et al. 2015). Folklorists certainly know about small groups and social interactions. This is just one area where folkloristics can contribute to the study of aging and in the development of elder services.

While some folklore discourse surrounding the work of elder arts may highlight the continuation of a tradition, it is important to note that not all expressive practices of older adults are continuation of traditions learned in an elder's youth. Geriatric psychiatrist Gene Cohen (1994) observed elders come to their creative practices in a variety of ways and times. Some elder artists, such as Charleston blacksmith Philip Simmons, continue to practice their craft throughout their lives, while others, such as memory painter Grandma Moses, might not begin their art-making practice until later in their life. An elder might also revive playing an instrument or making a craft that they may have learned as a child but not practiced in many years. This was the case with third-generation willow basketmaker LeRoy Graber, who at age ten learned to make baskets from his Mennonite grandfather. Years later, after retiring LeRoy revived the craft for which he would later receive a National Heritage Fellowship (Govenar n.d.). Cohen also observed that older adults may alter their creative practice in later life in a profound way. For example, woodcarver Bob Taylor had carved since he was eight years old but did not start carving scenes of his childhood until he retired from working as a patternmaker. He called these pieces his "memory carvings" (Kay 2016, 9–27) (fig. 0.3). Others may take up a creative practice after experiencing a rupture in their lives, such as the loss of a loved one. This was the case with my friend John Schoolman, who started making colorful walking sticks after his wife passed away (Kay 2016, 69–89). Many who work with elders recognize the benefit of creative practice for older adults, but more research is needed to better understand how these creative cultural expressions work in an elder's life, and whether it makes a difference in an older adult's life if a creative practice is maintained throughout one's life, adopted later, or revived from an earlier period (Ace et al. 2015).

## Folklorists and Elders

Since the founding of the field, folklorists have traveled far and wide to document cultural practices. Often their research led them to the oldest members of a community. In fact, younger scholars working with key elders is an established tradition in folklore: Alan Lomax and Huddie "Ledbelly" Ledbetter, Linda Dégh and Zsuzsanna Palko, Alan Jabbour and Henry Reed, or Henry Glassie and Hugh Nolan, to name a few folklorist-elder partnerships well known in the field. However, the foundational relationship between a young fieldworker and elder informant should not be taken lightly. As a fledgling scholar, I benefited greatly from a number of elders, who took me (an uninformed outsider) under their wing and taught me about the traditional ways of life in their community. Now as a midcareer scholar, I recognize the privilege that my youth afforded me when I first entered the field.

My initial experience with a grandparent-like interlocutor was in the summer of 1996; the Kentucky Folklife Program hired me to document traditional arts in the Cumberland Gap region. Working out of Pine Mountain State Resort Park in Pineville, Kentucky, I traveled the rural borderlands of Kentucky, Tennessee, and Virginia. I interviewed craftspeople such as white oak basketmaker Olen Cowen, bowl hewer James Miracle, and corn-shuck doll maker Mossy Muncy; I recorded folk songs and ballads from James Espen Honeycutt and old-time banjo tunes from Robert Hunley. In addition, I learned about folk medicine, traditional stories, and local foodways from several other area residents, most of whom were sixty or older. I cannot imagine a better field site for a novice folklore fieldworker or for a student wanting to learn about creative aging. Early that summer, local knife maker Sid Tibbs told me that I should talk to Damon Helton, a retired coal miner and willow furniture maker in Middlesboro, Kentucky. Sid went on to tell me that Damon probably wouldn't talk to me because I was an outsider and, worse yet, worked for the state park! He warned that Damon would probably run me off. A young fieldworker in my twenties, I was nervous about going to see Mr. Helton—but also curious.

I pulled into the drive. As I started to walk up to Mr. Helton's house, I saw the lanky older man grab something from his truck, which was parked in front of the house. He had a small pistol in his hand. My heart pounded. I said, "Mr. Helton, Sid Tibbs sent me. I am talking to people about local crafts and traditions." Instantly, he smiled and motioned me up to the porch. He told me the gun was for snakes, not folklorists. We spent the next three hours talking about gathering ginseng, building willow furniture, and harvesting hickory bark for chairs. He showed me a variety of keepsakes and mementos from his life in the region and shared their stories. He acted as if he had been waiting for me, or someone like me, to inquire about his life and his art. When it came time for me to leave, he seemed sorry that our time was up, so I said, "Do you mind if I come back by tomorrow, after I finish my other interviews?" He grinned and said, "Sure, buddy, come back tomorrow." I did go back the next day and a few times each week for the rest of the summer. For a few months, this retired coal miner adopted a college student; I occasionally helped him harvest willow (or "willers" as he called them) to make furniture, and he taught me about local life (fig. 0.4). When I was around, he often showed off his click-and-wheel, a small metal hoop he rolled with a stick, a toy like the one he played with in the coal camps of his youth. Damon knew about creative aging even though he never went to an arts class or participated in workshops by a certified teaching artist. He stayed vitally active and creatively engaged through practicing a variety of crafts and maintaining traditional practices that were rooted in his family and his community.

Why did Damon befriend a young stranger? Equally important, why did a fresh folklorist spend so much time learning esoteric information about local foodways, traditional medicine, and planting by the moon signs from this senior? Damon and I were engaged in an age-old practice of older adults passing on their knowledge to younger generations.[1] As Barbara Myerhoff (1984, 38) explained, "There are elderly people all over America, waiting only to be asked about their stories and folk art. Their memories and works are stored in boxes, in cellars, in trunks, in attics . . . needing only a witness to bring them to light, a recipi-

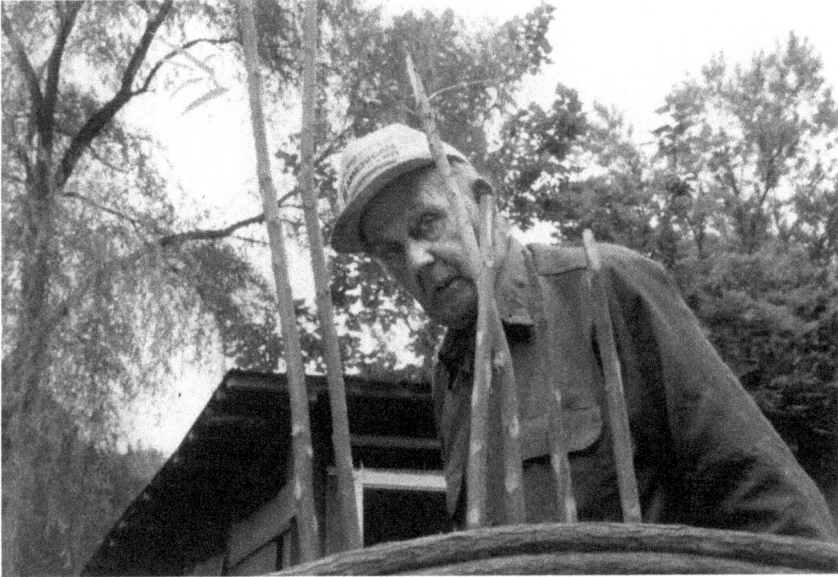

Fig. 0.4. Damon Helton making a willow love seat at his home in Middlesboro, Kentucky, 1996. *Photograph by Jon Kay.*

ent to complete the interchange that is requisite to all cultural transmission." It is exactly this role that I don't think folklorists and researchers have explored deeply enough. My job with the Kentucky Folklife Program that summer was to research the folklife of the region and produce a handful of public programs. Damon's job as an older adult was to pass on his knowledge, memories, and stories. What if my job in eastern Kentucky had not been to just document and present traditions but rather to understand how traditional arts support elders as they age and then to facilitate programs to support this work?

The passing on of traditional knowledge and skills can be seen as a special kind of generativity, a concept advanced by developmental psychologist Erik Erickson. He defined "generativity" as the "concern in establishing and guiding the next generation." Erickson (1950, 267) believed that this practice was an important developmental stage that often began in middle life and continue well into late adulthood. He and his wife, Joan, would later write that "old people can and need to maintain a *grand*-generative function" in their lives (Erikson and Erikson 1997, 63, emphasis original), which is what I had witnessed in the life of Damon Helton as well as elders at Rural Folklife Days. The passing on of intergenerational knowledge through a reciprocal relationship is a prime example of grand-generativity. The research and programming efforts of folklorists benefit

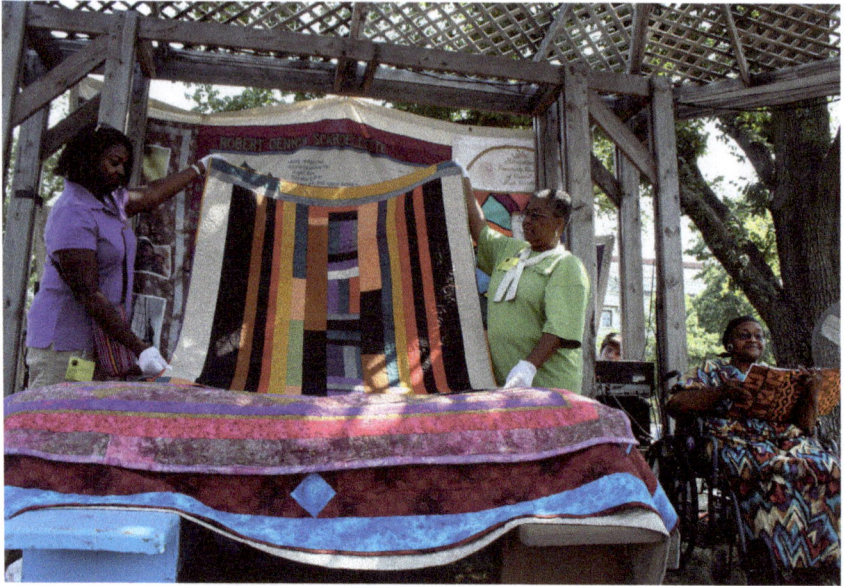

Fig. 0.5. Gladys Gorman Douglas leads a bed turning at the Smithsonian Folklife Festival, 2012. Janie Wyatt and Kathy Muhammad lift a quilt for the audience to see. *Courtesy of Traditional Arts Indiana.*

from local elders choosing to share their expertise and talents with us. Our older collaborators, however, often benefit as well from having us as their interlocutors, someone to "complete the interchange" that Myerhoff described.

Some older adults, such as Damon, express their generativity through close instruction, conversation, and mentorship that they may impart to a younger family member, neighbor, or other potential successor. In other settings, this interchange is broadcast to a larger group or shared at a public gathering, like at the Rural Folklife Days event. At these times, elders seize the stage and testify about their lives, values, and beliefs. In 2012, while working at the Smithsonian Folklife Festival, I hosted a traditional bed turning with the Sisters of the Cloth, an African American quilting guild from Fort Wayne, Indiana. A bed turning is a community ritual where layer upon layer of quilts are laid on a bed, and then one by one lifted up, and the story of each quilt's making or significance is shared. At this public turning, Gladys Gorman Douglas was the "storyteller of quilts." From her wheelchair, the septuagenarian addressed nearly a hundred festivalgoers who were there to see the quilts (fig. 0.5). However, Gladys broke with tradition and began by telling her life story, emphasizing how quiltmaking was an important part of her life and the African American experience. As she shared her life story and its connection to quilting, some of the other quilters got noticeably nervous at the length of her preamble. There were only forty-five minutes allotted to go through a thick stack of quilts and Gladys's storytelling was eating into this time. Finally, she brought her testimony to an end and proceeded to regale the audience with stories about the quilts that the Sisters had brought for the program.

Gladys recognized the significance of the program and the place; at that moment, an appreciative audience would listen to her. She knew the Smithsonian was recording her voice for the ages. On the National Mall—the place where Barack Obama took the oath of office and where Martin Luther King Jr. gave his "I Have a Dream" speech—Gladys Gorman Douglas spoke of her life as an African American woman and quilter. As a folklorist, I recognize that generativity flows in two directions. The stories and skills that pass to the next generation are an expression of an older adult's care for the future. Equally, however, an elder needs to feel their gifts are received. Both Gladys and Damon were lucky to find an appreciative audience for their knowledge and skills. Sadly, this is not true for all older adults.

## Folkloristics and Aging

Even though folklorists have often been the benefactors of the generativity of generous elders, we rarely take note of late adulthood as a significant time in the human life cycle where both creativity and the urge to share one's knowledge seem to flourish. While elderhood has not historically been an overt research topic in American folklore scholarship, the study of children's folklore has. In 1888 when the American Folklore Society was founded, children's traditions were flagged as a worthy topic of folkloristic inquiry (Newell 1888, 4). Nevertheless, there was no overt mention of the folklore of elders as a research focus. Why? Perhaps because the expressive acts of older adults were understood to be at the heart of most of our folklore scholarship. As the authors of *The Grand Generation* noted, "The field of folklore has been built from the memories of older people. . . . For centuries, classic collections of ballads and folktales, proverbs and riddles, and games and customs have been harvested from individuals who have lived long and remembered much" (Kirshenblatt-Gimblett et al. 2006, 32). By not recognizing the elderhood of our interlocutors, however, folklorists have left the expressive lives of older adults undertheorized and the application of our knowledge in this area underutilized. This collected volume encourages the development of folkloristic gerontology as an area of research, study, and practice in the field of folklore; nevertheless, the contributors are not the first to overtly study folklore and the expressive lives of older adults. As noted, folklorists researching the traditions, stories, and rituals of older adults is not new in American folkloristics. In fact, the 1970s and 1980s witnessed a blossoming of studies about folklore and aging.

The work of Barbara Myerhoff is often referenced as the foundation of much of the folkloristic research of the expressive lives of elders. A visual anthropologist, Myerhoff conducted ethnographic research with older Jewish immigrants living in Venice, California. Her book *Number Our Days* probes the celebrations, rituals, and everyday interactions of elders at the Aliyah Senior Citizens' Center. Before becoming a book, Myerhoff's research with this group was featured in a television documentary also named *Number Our Days*, which received the 1976 Academy Award for best short documentary. In the book, she explains that "reviewing one's life and reminiscing, much practiced by the very old, are expressions of their attempts to find themselves to be the same person throughout the life cycle"—highlighting not just the cultural aspects of their expressive acts but also the psychological work that narratives and rituals play in the lives of elders (Myerhoff 1979, 108).

Myerhoff's writings inspired a generation of folklorists and anthropologists to study aging. Much of the work done by folklorists in the 1980s and 1990s, however, was produced not in the academy but rather in the public sector. For example, alongside the occupational traditions of Alaska and "Black American Urban Culture," the 1984 Festival of American Folklife presented the life-story projects of older adults who recalled their former lives through stories and art. Vilius Variakojis of Chicago shared dioramas that he made to resemble the Lithuanian village of his youth, Ethel Mohamed showed her embroidery that revealed scenes from her family life and personal history, and Elijah Pierce told the stories cut in his woodcarvings (Hufford 1984, 32–35). That same year, Mary Hufford, Marjorie Hunt, and Steven Zeitlin produced *The Grand Generation: Memory, Mastery, Legacy*, a Smithsonian exhibition with an accompanying book (1984) and documentary film (1987), which explored memory projects, creative practices, and life stories as significant tools for elders. At the 2017 Meeting of the American Folklore Society, a panel marked the thirtieth anniversary of *The Grand Generation* book, noting the significance of the project and how it was at the vanguard of research into creative aging. It was so ahead of its time that in 2006, almost twenty years after its original publication, the American Society on Aging republished the book's introductory essay in their journal *Generations*. Folklorists were ahead of the curve in recognizing the value of creative practice in the lives of older adults. In 1984, Bess Lomax Hawes, the director of the National Endowment for the Arts' Folk and Traditional Arts Program from 1977 to 1992, observed that "so much of the gerontological literature . . . treats the elderly as a problem and old age as a time of life when a burdensome series of special conditions have to be met." She contrasted that position by stating that in the folk arts, older adults are "thought of as the solution" (Hawes 1984, 31). Folklorists recognize that communities often rely on elders as the keepers and teachers of important community knowledge and traditional practices.

Where Myerhoff's work encouraged a range of academic studies in aging, Alan Jabbour seems to have been the first to suggest a direct applied folklore approach to traditional arts and aging. The former director of the National Endowment for the Arts' Folk and Traditional Arts Program and the Library of Congress's American Folklife Center, Jabbour moved beyond documenting these expressive acts. He rightly recognized that traditional arts could be leveraged to improve the quality of life of older adults. He advised that arts interventions in eldercare work best when they are culturally grounded. Writing about the role of traditional arts in aging, Jabbour noted that there is no universal artistic therapy that could be taught or administered to older adults, but rather, tapping into the power of "folk arts means fundamentally drawing out special forms of expression people already possess, not laying on arts, forms, or programs they lack"(1981, 143). I believe that Jabbour's observation is the foundation of a folkloristic approach to gerontology—arts and aging therapies work best when they align with an individual's personal and cultural identity.

As referenced above, folklorists working in the public sector in the 1980s and 1990s began researching, developing exhibitions about, and presenting programs on the expressive lives of older adults (Beck 1982; Hufford 1984; Hufford, Hunt, and Zeitlin 1987; Yocom 1994). Following Myerhoff's example, folklorists produced several documentary films about aging tradition bearers and artists. An example is *Water from Another Time* (1982) directed by folklorist Dillon Bustin and filmmaker Richard Kane. It follows Bustin as he interacts with old-time fiddler Lotus Dickey, tinkerer Elmer Boyd, and folk painter Lois Doane. This film deftly demonstrates how skills, stories, and habits developed in one's youth can help an elder age well.

By screening films such as *The Grand Generation* and *Water from Another Time*, folklorist David Shuldiner developed a robust arts-in-aging initiative through his work with the Connecticut Humanities Council. As one of the pioneers of applied folklore and aging, Shuldiner worked with the Connecticut State Department of Aging to facilitate programs and listen to life stories of elders throughout the state. In 1994, he reported on his gerontological work in his essay "Promoting Self-Worth among the Aging," in which he suggested that there was a role for public folklorists in facilitating life-review and life-story telling as a way to improve the quality of life of older adults (Shuldiner 1994, 217).[2] Unfortunately, few folklorists followed him into applied folklore and aging work.

While much of the scholarship on traditional art and aging grew out of work produced in public arts and humanities organizations, scholars in the academy also took up research into late-life creativity, storytelling, and the traditional art practices of elders. Simon Bronner's (1985) *Chain Carvers* explored how the carving projects of older men help them cope with many of the hardships of aging. Similarly, Patrick Mullen's (1992) *Listening to Old Voices* links reminiscence and life-review scholarship to folklore by applying Robert J. Havighurst's concept of "successful aging" and Robert Butler's positive perspective of reminiscence to his study of folklore in the lives of elders.[3] Although relatively brief and published in an undergraduate textbook, Barbara Kirshenblatt-Gimblett's (1989) "Objects of Memory: Material Culture as Life Review" amplified Hufford, Hunt, and Zeitlin's work on memory objects in later life. In 2007, Kirshenblatt-Gimblett revisited this topic in *They Called Me Mayer July* (2007), which focuses on the memory paintings of Kirshenblatt-Gimblett's father, Mayer Kirshenblatt. This collaborative work marries the senior's images and stories about the Jewish community in Apt (Opatów), Poland, with a thoughtful analysis by his daughter, resulting in a very personal and insightful study into life-story art. Each of these scholars working in the academy recognized the importance of narrative and other forms of expressive culture to the aging process.

As university-based folklorists researched the narrative and creative practices of seniors, public folklorist began applying their research to the design of new arts-based programs for older adults. In the late 1990s, the North Dakota Arts Council (NDAC) undertook a project to use traditional arts to improve the quality of life of residents in assisted-living facilities throughout the state. Since then, the NDAC and North Dakota state folklorist Troyd Geist have grown and developed their "Art for Life Program," which works with arts agencies, elder-care facilities, and folk artists to improve the health and wellness of older adults through interactive arts programs. In 2017, the NDAC published *Sundogs and Sunflowers: An Art for Life Program Guide for Creative Aging, Health, and Wellness* (Geist 2017).[4] In addition to North Dakota's groundbreaking work, Kathleen Mundell coordinated the Creative Aging Program of the Maine Arts Commission (MAC) that demonstrated the importance of creative engagement for older adults. She linked the program with the MAC Traditional Arts Apprenticeship Program with great success (Mundell 2015). Since then, she has developed an "Elderhood Arts" program, which honors elders as keepers of family and community culture. While other folk arts programs have also done arts in aging work, Geist and Mundell have been leaders in the development of public creative aging programs based on the traditional arts. From Hufford, Hunt, and Zeitlin's *The Grand Generation* to Geist's Art for Life Program, some folklorists have studied and promoted culturally relevant creative aging practices; however, folklorists in general usually view aging studies as a secondary focus in their research and programs. What would the field of folklore look like if more folklorists made aging the central concern of their work?

## Folkloristic Gerontology

In 1998, David Hufford (1998, 296–97) extended an invitation asking folklorists to follow him into the realm of applied folklore and health, a domain in which he had productively worked. Despite his compelling description of the field, few joined him in working in applied health settings. Since publishing *Folk Art and Aging*, I have worked with gerontologists, therapists, and eldercare professionals, and as a whole, they are interested in the observations, interpretations, and methods of folklore; however, folkloristic gerontology is underdeveloped and undertheorized. This edited volume encourages folklorists to turn their folklore and ethnographic skills toward researching and documenting the expressive lives of older adults. Folklorists can leverage their disciplinary theories, methods, and training, as well as their ethnographic observations to improve the quality of life of older adults. This book is not a comprehensive study of vernacular forms of creative aging; neither is it a how-to guide for folklore and aging practice—that would be premature. Rather, it gathers the observations of folklorists working with older adults and provides a glimpse of this proposed field of folkloristic gerontology.

Gerontology is the study of the aging process and the problems associated with it, usually with an eye toward understanding and improving the lives of older adults. Some gerontologists are therapists or social workers, while others are medical professionals. In general, the term *gerontology* gathers together a range of professional activities aimed at studying and serving older adults. In the 1980s, folklorist Kenneth Goldstein served as the chairman of the Social Gerontology program at the University of Pennsylvania. He had developed an interest in gerontology through his work with elder informants as well as from the projects of his students, Hufford, Hunt, and Zeitlin.[5] Goldstein recognized the potential of applied folklore to the service of health and wellness for older adults.

I offer "folkloristic gerontology" as a subfield in aging studies that marshals the theories, methods, and practices of folklore to the research of and service to older adults. From folklore's scholarly research with older tradition bearers to their public programs with master folk artists, folklorists have a working knowledge of folklore and aging. Consider the Heritage Fellowships of the National Endowment for the Arts. This program honors master traditional artists whose music, dance, and craft are rooted in community life. Although not a requirement, most of the recipients are in their seventies, eighties, and nineties, and a major factor in their selection is generativity—are they passing on their traditional knowledge to the next generation? This important national program amplifies the image of older adults as central agents in their communities and as essential artists and knowledge bearers. Similarly, most state folk arts agencies have apprenticeship programs that support master artists in the passing on of traditional knowledge and skills to an apprentice—a program that codifies Erikson's notion of generativity. While these programs may not be framed as folkloristic gerontology projects, they do point toward the range of skills and competencies that folklorists possess that could be deployed to support the research of and services to older adults. While Geist and Mundell have developed public and

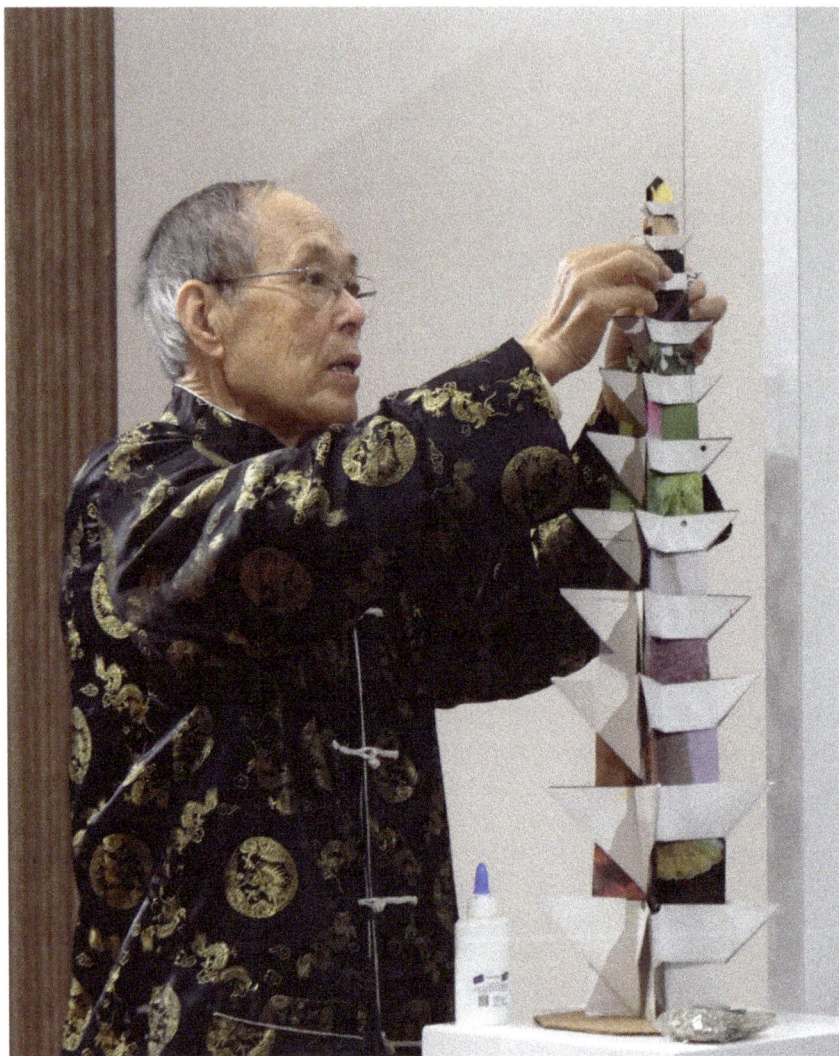

Fig. 0.6. James Min-Ching Yang builds a paper pagoda for the "Creative Aging" exhibition at the Mathers Museum of World Cultures, 2018. *Courtesy of the Mathers Museum of World Cultures, Indiana University, Bloomington.*

applied folklore models for traditional arts and creative aging services, I believe their work can be replicated and expanded, and new models developed. While this volume centers on the material culture practices of older adults, folkloristic gerontology could concentrate on a range of expressive and communicative behavior that would include the oral, material, musical, or customary aspects of an elder's everyday life (fig. 0.6).

I recently curated an exhibition at the Mathers Museum of World Cultures centered on the creative pursuits of older adults in Indiana. I included artists such as woodcarver Bob Taylor and rug maker Marian Sykes, both of whom were featured in my book *Folk Art and Aging*. I also invited other older artists whose creative practices coupled life review and storytelling with art making. The work of James Min-Ching Yang, a Chinese calligrapher and musician, was also included in the exhibition. One day, he came to the museum to serve as an artist in residence at the museum and to teach Chinese paper folding to my Indiana Folklore class. He had absorbed the craft many years ago; in fact, so long ago he couldn't even remember when he had learned it. It seemed as if he had always known how to fold paper birds and pagodas. James loved teaching the students, and the students soaked up his instruction. The lesson for the day may have seemed as if it was paper folding, but really, it was a class about generativity. As a class, we discussed the process of sharing knowledge and receiving instruction from elders. Facilitating this intergenerational exchange was incredibly rewarding for the students, James, as well as for me. As we walked through the exhibit after the class, he stood in the gallery where several of his pieces of calligraphy and a few folded pagodas were on display. He paused and looked at me. "This is my place," he said. "When I get back from Taiwan, I will come and sit here and play erhu." The Chinese bowed instrument stirs strong emotions for the elder, and his willingness to return to the museum and share his talents is revealing. What if folklorists worked to help produce spaces where older adults could come, create, and share their talents? Perhaps there is a role for folkloristic gerontologists to work with community museums, senior centers, public libraries, and assisted-living facilities to create these opportunities and experiences for elders.

Another area where folklorists can contribute to the support of seniors is in the facilitation of life storytelling—that is, creating opportunities for elders to share meaningful personal experience narratives with others. The use of life history and life story is a popular therapy for older adults. However, folklore's attention to the dialogical and performative aspects of narration, I believe, could add much to this work. While our field has deep roots in the study of stories, it is our attention to context and performance that allows us to understand the dynamic life story work of older adults—and how the telling and retelling of personal experience narratives function in the lives of elders. In addition to research into life stories, there is much work to be done in facilitating the telling of life stories. I have collected narratives from several elders after they were diagnosed with a terminal disease. Often they are looking for a receptive listener, a witness to record their stories, someone to ask them about their life and its meaning, and a way to leave a legacy.

Another area of research and programming might be in foodways. From educational lesson plans to culinary tourism, folklorists have developed approaches, skills, and programs related to food production, preparation, and preservation (Brown and Mussell 1984; Humphrey and Humphrey 1991; Long 2015; Wilson and Gillespie 1999). A recent study explored the relationship between food activities and the maintenance of elder identity. The authors of the study noted that while nutrition and food access may present real concerns for many elders, there are other food-related factors that must be considered, such as "how food activities contribute to psychological well-being in later life" (Plastow, Atwal, and Gilhooly 2015). For example, food production and preparation are important for many older adults as they construct and maintain their sense of self, which is explored more fully in Christensen's essay in this volume.

## Resilience and Adaptability in Later Life

From the stories we tell and the music we make, to the foods we prepare and the things we create, folklore is our adaptive repertoire for dealing with our everyday encounters and problems. They are not the ephemera of our culture but rather our creative core, our cultural competency for handling whatever life may throw at us. Developmental psychologists Paul and Margret Baltes (1990) offered a successful-aging model that conceived of an adaptive process by which elders select an aspect of their life which they then optimize to maximize the gains and compensate for loses that they may experience as they age. From woodcarving and quiltmaking to cooking and storytelling, these cultivated life domains often include expressive forms that help elders age positively. Furthermore, a 2016 study found that older adults who frequently discussed their adaptive strategies and compensations often experienced a high degree of well-being even though they may have low physical function (Carpentieri et al. 2017).

In my research into the expressive lives of older adults, I have seen the importance of adaptability and resilience in the maintenance and recovery of an elder's quality of life. The concept of resilience, however, is often oversimplified: "Oh, she is so resilient. I could never do that," one might say. Resilience is not a singular thing to have, however, but rather a system of supports used by people to address the physical, social, and psychological strains that may potentially disrupt their everyday lives. Psychologists Ursula M. Staudinger and Werner Greve (2015, 1) define resilience as "a constellation of risk factors or stressors on the one hand and of available protective factors that are both of a psychological and non-psychological nature, on the other." Traditional arts, narrative practices, and other expressive acts are noteworthy "protective factors" in the lives of older adults. Many folklorists have witnessed how cultural practices such as crafts, music, games, and traditional foods help elders retain or recover functionality

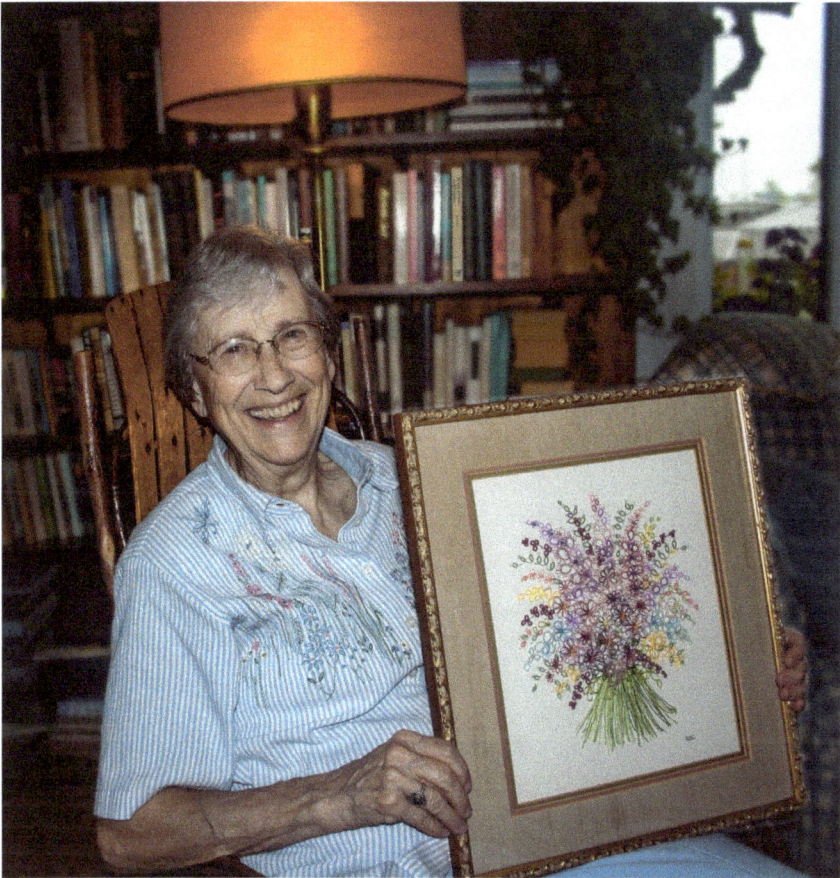

Fig. 0.7. Ruth Neuhouser with a tatted-lace flower arrangement, Upland, Indiana, 2009. *Courtesy of Traditional Arts Indiana.*

after a physical, social, or psychological event interrupted their life. Although making a quilt, playing an accordion, or euchring an opponent with a deck of cards may not cure heart disease, diabetes, or arthritis, it may help heal an older adult as they strive to regain control in their lives after a major life event.

For many, a traditional art or cultural practice serves as a personal anchor when hardships and difficulties emerge in later life. When, due to declining mobility, Ruth Neuhouser could no longer work in the flowerbeds that surrounded her home in Upland, Indiana, a new art form emerged (fig. 0.7). Tatting, a craft she learned as a child, blossomed in her later years. She started knotting intricate lace flowers, which she then would artfully arrange into beautiful bouquets

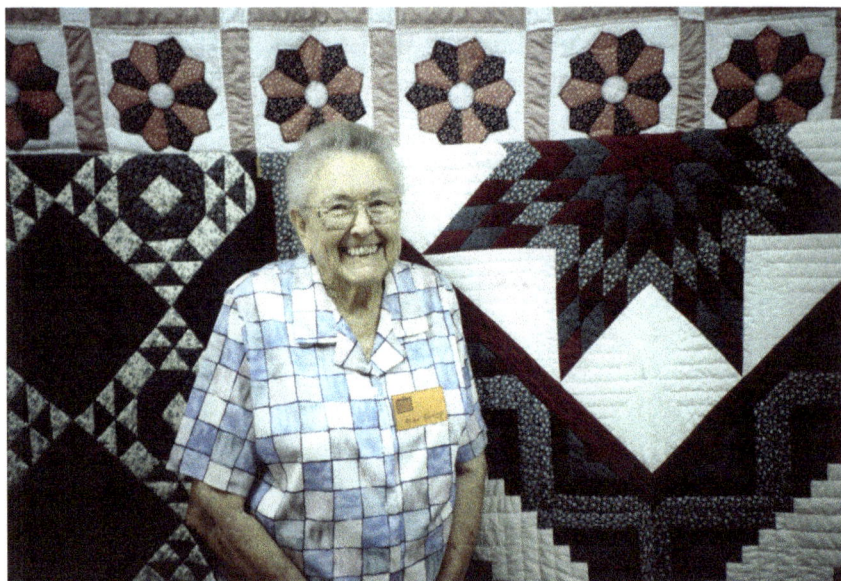

Fig. 0.8. Quilter Nancy Morgan at Rural Folklife Days event at the Stephen Foster Folk Culture Center in White Springs, Florida, 1999. *Photograph by Jon Kay.*

reminiscent of the ones she cut from her gardens (fig. 0.7). When arthritis made it difficult for Nancy Morgan of White Springs, Florida, to work at the quilting frame with her friends, she revived the art of briar stitching, a craft remembered from her childhood (fig. 0.8). Using thick thread to embroider flowers, birds, and turkey tracks into randomly pieced fabric, Nancy made several crazy quilts and wall hangings for friends and family. For both Nancy and Ruth, their adaptive art allowed them to maintain their sense of well-being and regain meaning in their lives, even when physical factors restricted their creative options.

A more striking example of resiliency in later life is the story of celebrated baker Mary Alice Collins, who each year would win dozens of ribbons at the Indiana State Fair for the pies that she made. Traditional Arts Indiana, the program I direct, honored her as a 2014 Indiana State Fair Master for her fifty-plus years of participation at the fair. Two years later, Mary Alice became gravely ill; all of her fingers as well as both legs were amputated to save her life. Nevertheless, the following summer, she entered more than thirty pies in the fair, and each year since. Why? Competitive baking allowed her to demonstrate to herself and others that she could adapt to her new life. This is not to say that baking pies, quilting, or lacemaking makes life easy but rather that the maintaining, reviving, acquiring, or adapting of an expressive practice provides an older adult with an additional resource that they can employ when they are faced with a seemingly insurmountable stress on their life.

Not only do the traditional arts and expressive practices of older adults help when elders face the tribulations that so often accompany advanced age, but they also often revive, adopt, or invent new creative practices as a strategy for addressing late-life hardships. The authors of *The Grand Generation* observed that many of the elderly artists featured in their exhibition about late-life creativity started, revived, or translated their creative practice when their lives were disrupted by a stressful life event "that abruptly severed them from the world as they knew it." These expressive practices worked to "minimize the fissures created when the people or things on which life depended have suddenly disappeared" (Hufford, Hunt, and Zeitlin 1987, 43–44). As folklorists have noted, people deploy folklore as a coping strategy to make sense out of chaos. From the HIV/AIDS epidemic to Hurricane Katrina, survivors use stories, art, music, food, and other expressive forms to restore order and come to a new understanding of their lives (Ancelet, Lindahl, and Gaudet 2013; Lindahl 2006; Wells 2012).

While expressive practices provide a mitigating resource for older adults when they face struggles in their lives, approaching the practices with adaptability is central to finding fulfillment after a life-changing event. Where Nancy Morgan and Ruth Neuhouser had to modify their creative practices in order to sustain satisfaction in their lives and their work, Mary Alice Collins had to alter her approach to her work, often relying on her husband, Darl, for specific tasks, such as weaving the artfully latticed tops to her fruit pies. The couple always worked together to produce the pies for the fair, but just as baking was a resource that Mary Alice could draw upon to sustain her, so was the support and help of her husband (Duncan 2016). Traditional arts and other forms of folklore are not silver bullets for health and wellness in later life—far from it. Rather, they are points of light within that constellation of resources identified by Staudinger and Greve that older adults can draw upon as they negotiate a new understanding of and satisfaction with their lives.

In *Chain Carvers*, Simon Bronner (1985) noted that physical, psychological, and social stresses prompted the older men in his book to take up carving again. Carving was an adaptive practice that helped the retirees cope with their changing lives and relationships. Similarly, in my book *Folk Art and Aging* (Kay 2016), I show how art making—specifically, the memory projects of older adults—serves as an adaptive strategy for their makers after they retire, lose a loved one, become dislocated from their home, or some other physical or psychological strain is placed on their lives. The work that these everyday practices do in the lives of older adults, however, is often trivialized—after all, her quilting is just a hobby, that painting is not very pretty, or your music is not commercially viable. As craft scholar Allen Eaton (1937, 9) observed, however, the time has come "when every kind of work will be judged by two measurements: one by the product itself, as is now done, the other by the effect of the work on the producer. When that time comes the handicrafts will be given a much more important place in our plan of living than they now have, for unquestionably they possess values which are not generally recognized."

Using ethnographic methods, folklorists can shed light on the complex work that expressive practices play in the lives of older adults, especially in the area of maintaining or regaining one's quality of life in later years.

Independent of folklore scholarship, gerontologists are beginning to recognize the special role traditional arts can play in the lives of older adults. Studying the function of traditional arts in the lives of older women in Crete, occupational therapist Despina Tzanidaki and Francis Reynolds (2011, 375) noted that the participants in their study "gained status, and a culturally recognized role in the community, from preserving and transmitting the skills required for indigenous forms of art and craft work." This observation may seem fairly obvious to folklorists, but the fact that other scholars studying aging recognize the unique role that traditional arts play in the lives of elders is noteworthy. Because of the way grants are made in the arts in the United States, traditional arts are often viewed as a separate genre of creative practice. Folk arts are often conceived of as a category on the same level as music, dance, or craft. However, "folk arts" are not a parallel genre of art but rather refer to the way creative practices are culturally and socially rooted in individual and community life. While it is true that the arts in general can improve the health and wellness of older adults, culturally and personally relevant expressive endeavors may hold even greater potential for helping elders age well.[6]

By 2020, people aged sixty-five and older will outnumber children under the age of five for the first time in human history (He, Goodkind, and Kowal 2016, 3). By 2050, the population in the United States aged sixty-five and older is projected to be 83.7 million, nearly double current population estimates (Ortman, Velkoff, and Hogan 2014). Is the field of folklore study ready for the cultural changes that lie ahead? It is my hope that this edited volume will not only ignite serious conversations about folklore and aging in general but also specifically develop a set of folklore theories and methods that can be applied to aging studies, encourage research into effective models of folk arts programs in eldercare settings, revive folkloristic interest in life review work, and develop a skills set and competencies that might lead to a field of folkloristic gerontology. From boot making and quilting to woodcarving and canning, the chapters that follow explore the expressive lives of older adults and provide a glimpse into folklore and aging. They focus on the material culture practices of elders and the ways that folklorists can contribute to the study of aging. Some of the essays are descriptive in nature, providing a snapshot of the creative lives of older adults; others engage with the evidence-based studies of gerontologists and related scholars, while a third group outlines the methods employed by folklorists who are working in applied arts and aging settings.

JON KAY is Clinical Associate Professor in the Department of Folklore and Ethnomusicology at Indiana University and Director of Traditional Arts Indiana at the Mathers Museum of World Cultures. He is author of *Folk Art and Aging: Life-Story Objects and Their Makers* (IUP).

## Works Cited

Ace Everett, Gay Hanna, Janice Blanchard, Judith-Kate Friedman, Judy Rollins, Linda No-
    elker, Paula Cleggett, and Tobi Abramson. 2016. *The Summit on Creativity and Aging
    in America*. White House Conference on Aging. http://www.issuelab.org/permalink
    /resource/23933.
Ancelet, Barry Jean, Carl Lindahl, and Marcia Gaudet. 2013. *Second Line Rescue: Impro-
    vised Responses to Katrina and Rita*. Jackson: University Press of Mississippi.
Baltes, Paul B., and Margret M. Baltes. 1990. "Psychological Perspectives on Successful Ag-
    ing: The Model of Selective Optimization with Compensation." In *Successful Aging:
    Perspectives from the Behavioral Sciences*, edited by Paul B. Baltes and Margret M.
    Baltes, 1–34. Cambridge: Cambridge University Press.
Bauman, Richard. 1972. "Differential Identity and the Social Base of Folklore." In *Toward
    New Perspectives in Folklore*, edited by Americo Parédes and Richard Bauman, 31–41.
    Publication Series of the American Folklore Society, Bibliographical and Special
    Series (23). Austin: University of Texas Press.
Beck, Jane C. 1982. *Always in Season: Folk Art and Traditional Culture in Vermont: Ver-
    mont Historical Society Museum, Montpelier, 8.5.-1.11.1982* . . . Montpelier: Vermont
    Council on the Arts.
Ben-Amos, Dan. 1972. "Toward a Definition of Folklore in Context." In *Toward New Per-
    spectives in Folklore*, edited by Americo Parédes and Richard Bauman, 3–15. Publica-
    tion Series of the American Folklore Society, Bibliographical and Special Series (23).
    Austin: University of Texas Press.
Bronner, Simon J. 1985. *Chain Carvers: Old Men Crafting Meaning*. Lexington: University
    Press of Kentucky.
Brown, Linda Keller, and Kay Mussell, eds. 1984. *Ethnic and Regional Foodways in the
    United States: Performance of Group Identity*. Knoxville: University of Tennessee
    Press.
Bustin, Dillon, and Richard Kane, dirs. 1982. *Water from Another Time*. Watertown, MA:
    Documentary Educational Resources. https://www.kanopy.com/wayf/product/water
    -another-time-1982.
Butler, Robert. 1963. "The Life Review: An Interpretation of Reminiscence in the Aged."
    *Psychiatry* 26 (1): 65–76.
Carpentieri, Jon D., Jane Elliott, Caroline E. Brett, and Ian J. Deary. 2017. "Adapting to
    Aging: Older People Talk about Their Use of Selection, Optimization, and Compen-

sation to Maximize Well-Being in the Context of Physical Decline." *The Journals of Gerontology: Series B* 72 (2): 351–61. https://doi.org/10.1093/geronb/gbw132.

Cohen, Gene D. 1994. "Creativity and Aging: Relevance to Research, Practice, and Policy." *American Journal of Geriatric Psychiatry* 2 (4): 277–81.

Doucette, Laurel Catherine. 1986. *The Emergence of New Expressive Skills in Retirement and Later Life in Contemporary Newfoundland*. PhD diss., Memorial University of Newfoundland.

Duncan, Mallory. 2016. "Award-Winning Baker Overcomes Challenges to Compete at Indiana State Fair." *WISH*, August 12, 2016. www.wishtv.com/news/local-news/award -winning-baker-overcomes-challenges-to-compete-at-indiana-state-fair_ 20180412011509613/1116365757.

Eaton, Allen. 1937. "The Rural Arts Exhibition." An Exhibition of the Rural Arts Held in Connection with the 75th Anniversary of the Founding of the Department of Agriculture, 1862–1937, November 14–30, 1937, in the patio of the Administration Building of the US Department of Agriculture. https://hdl.handle.net/2027 /coo.31924014091924.

Erikson, Erik H. 1950. *Childhood and Society*. New York: Norton.

Erikson, Erik H., and Joan M. Erikson. 1997. *The Life Cycle Completed: Extended Version with New Chapters on the Ninth Stage of Development*. New York: Norton.

Geist, Troyd A. 2017. *Sundogs and Sunflowers: An Art for Life Program Guide for Creative Aging, Health, and Wellness*. Bismarck: North Dakota Council on the Arts.

Govenar, Alan, ed. n.d. "LeRoy Graber." Masters of Traditional Arts. Accessed April 15, 2018. http://www.mastersoftraditionalarts.org/artists/116.

Hawes, Bess Lomax. 1984. "Folk Arts and the Elderly." In *Festival of American Folklife Program Book*, edited by T. Vennum, 29–31. Washington, DC: Smithsonian Institution.

He, Wan, Daniel Goodkind, and Paul R. Kowal. 2016. *An Aging World: International Population Reports*. Washington, DC: US Department of Health and Human Services National Institutes of Health/ National Institute on Aging. http://cdn.cnsnews.com /attachments/census_bureau-an_aging_world-2015.pdf.

Holt-Lunstad, Julianne, et al. 2015. "Loneliness and Social Isolation as Risk Factors for Mortality." *Perspectives on Psychological Science* 10 (2): 227–37. doi:10.1177 /1745691614568352.

Hufford, David. 1998. "Folklore Studies Applied to Health." *Journal of Folklore Research* 353 (3): 295–313.

Hufford, Mary. 1984. "All of Life's a Stage: The Aesthetics of Life Review." In *Festival of American Folklife Program Book*, edited by T. Vennum, 32–35. Washington, DC: Smithsonian Institution.

Hufford, Mary, Marjorie Hunt, and Steven Zeitlin. 1987. *The Grand Generation: Memory, Mastery, Legacy*. Washington, DC: Smithsonian Institution.

Humphrey, Theodore C., and Lin T. Humphrey. 1991. *We Gather Together: Food and Festival in American Life*. Logan: Utah State University Press.

Jabbour, Alan. 1981. "Some Thoughts from a Folk Cultural Perspective." In *Perspectives on Aging: Exploding the Myths*, edited by Priscilla W. Johnston, 139–49. Cambridge, MA: Ballinger.

Kay, Jon. 2016. *Folk Art and Aging: Life-Story Objects and Their Makers*. Bloomington: Indiana University Press. https://scholarworks.iu.edu/dspace/handle/2022/20906.

Kirshenblatt-Gimblett, Barbara. 1989. "Objects of Memory: Material Culture as Life Review." In *Folk Groups and Folklore Genres: A Reader*, edited by Elliott Oring, 329–38. Logan: Utah State University Press.

Kirshenblatt-Gimblett, Barbara, Mary Hufford, Marjorie Hunt, and Steve Zeitlin. 2006. "The Grand Generation: Folklore and the Culture of Aging." *Generations* 1 (Spring): 32–37.

Kirshenblatt, Mayer, and Barbara Kirshenblatt-Gimblett. 2007. *They Called Me Mayer July: Painted Memories of a Jewish Childhood in Poland before the Holocaust*. Berkeley: University of California Press.

Lindahl, Carl. 2006. "Storms of Memory: New Orleanians Surviving Katrina in Houston." *Callaloo* 29 (4): 1526–38. http://www.jstor.org.proxyiub.uits.iu.edu/stable/4488495.

Long, Lucy M. 2015. *The Food and Folklore Reader*. London: Bloomsbury Academic.

Mundell, Kathleen. 2015. "Creativity and Aging." *Maine Policy Review* 24 (2): 76–79.

Mullen, Patrick Borden. 1992. *Listening to Old Voices: Folklore, Life Stories, and the Elderly*. Urbana: University of Illinois Press.

Myerhoff, Barbara G. 1979. *Number Our Days*. New York: Dutton.

———. 1984. "Life Not Death in Venice." In *Festival of American Folklife Program Book*, edited by T. Vennum. Washington, DC: Smithsonian Institution.

Newell, William Wells. 1888. On the Field and Work of a Journal of American Folklore." *Journal of American Folklore* 1 (1): 3–7.

Ortman, Jennifer M., Victoria A. Velkoff, and Howard Hogan. 2014. *An Aging Nation: The Older Population in the United States*. http://www.census.gov/prod/2014pubs /p25–1140.pdf.

Plastow, Nicola Ann, Anita Atwal, and Mary Gilhooly. 2015. "Food Activities and Identity Maintenance in Old Age: A Systematic Review and Meta-Synthesis." *Aging & Mental Health* 19 (8): 667–78.

Rowe, John W., and Robert L. Kahn. 1997. "Successful Aging." *The Gerontologist* 37 (4): 433–40.

Shuldiner, David P. 1994. "Promoting Self-Worth among the Aging." In *Putting Folklore to Use*, edited by Michael Owen Jones, 214–25. Lexington: University of Kentucky Press.

———. 1997. *Folklore, Culture, and Aging: A Research Guide*. Westport, CT: Greenwood.

Staudinger, Ursula M., and Werner Greve. 2015. "Resilience and Aging." In *Encyclopedia of Geropsychology*, edited by Nancy A. Pachana. Accessed November 20, 2017. http:// www.ursulastaudinger.com/wp-content/uploads/2017/08/Stauger-Greve-Resilience -and-Aging2015.pdf.

Tzanidaki, Despina, and Francis Reynolds. 2011. "Exploring the Meanings of Making Traditional Arts and Crafts among Older Women in Crete, Using Interpretative Phenomenological Analysis." *British Journal of Occupational Therapy* 74 (8): 375–82.

Wells, Kate. 2012. *Siyazama: Art, AIDS, and Education in South Africa*. Scottsville, South Africa: University of KwaZulu-Natal Press.

Wilson, David Scofield, and Angus K. Gillespie. 1999. *Rooted in America Foodlore of Popular Fruits and Vegetables*. Knoxville: University of Tennessee Press.

Yale, Stacy Lundin. 2004. "Aging in Eden: Reframing Treatment Paradigms for Elderly Patients." *Alternative and Complementary Therapies* 9 (1): 42–44.

Yocom, Margaret R., ed. 1994. *Logging in the Maine Woods: The Paintings of Alden Grant*. Rangeley, ME: Rangeley Lakes Region Logging Museum.

## Notes

1. I was not unique in Damon's sharing of traditional knowledge and time. The widower often watched his grandchildren and actively tried to pass on his knowledge and skill to them.

2. Shuldiner (1997) also compiled a thorough research guide about folklore and aging, which includes a valuable annotated bibliography of articles, books, and films.

3. A relative concept, the idea of "successful aging" is based on the premise that seniors need to find satisfaction in/with their lives, which includes both their memories and their current life situation (Rowe and Kahn 1997). Robert Butler's 1963 article "The Life Review" transformed the scholarly and therapeutic understanding of reminiscence and life review. He argued that the act of reviewing one's life is a "naturally occurring, universal mental process" (1963, 66).

4. Both Geist and Mundell report in more detail about their traditional arts and aging initiatives in later chapters in this volume.

5. Recognizing the potential of applied folklore research and methods, Goldstein was also intrigued by Laurel Doucette's (1985) doctoral dissertation, *The Emergence of New Expressive Skills in Retirement and Later Life in Contemporary Newfoundland*. Doucette (1985, iii) noted that "in restricting their attention to the elderly in their role as tradition bearers," folklorists had overlooked several recurring themes in the expressive practices of older adults: autobiography, integration, the preparation of cultural legacy, status maintenance and enhancement, play, compensation, social and cultural involvement, and the creation of a personal domain.

6. For more about creative aging, see *The Summit on Creativity and Aging in America* (Ace et al. 2016).

# Part I
# Observations on
# Folklore and Aging

# 1      Boot Lasts and Basket Lists

## *Joe Patrickus's Customized Art and Life*

### Lisa L. Higgins

In 2006, PSYCHOLOGIST and gerontologist Gene D. Cohen published his re-search team's landmark multiyear creativity and aging study, which not only examined the benefits of "cultural programs" on "older adults" but also defined the "creative aging" movement. Cohen's team included Susan Perlstein, who founded the National Center for Creative Aging in 2001. Cohen and his team's work boosted new research, funding opportunities, projects, and collaboration between organizations. A national movement launched in gerontology and the arts (Cohen et al. 2006).

The Missouri Arts Council became a leader in the new movement and par-ticipated in a 2013 pilot project funded by the National Endowment for the Arts. Creative Aging Program specialist Virginia Sanders identified Missouri individ-uals and organizations whose projects fit definitions of "creative aging." Sanders also immediately recognized that our state's folk arts projects (and those in our sister states) have promoted cross-generational and lifelong artistic participa-tion and learning for decades. The Missouri Arts Council then established the Creative Aging Network, forging relationships with project managers, artists, researchers, and educators and fostering participation in theater, film, and dance projects for "mature" Missourians.

In the midst of this movement, with eighteen years of anecdotal evidence as the director of the Missouri Folk Arts Program, I grew cognizant of the positive impacts of traditional arts on the elders who participate in our projects. During this same time frame, folklore colleagues Troyd Geist and Jon Kay conducted ethnographic research and engaged artists in "arts and aging" projects in North

*The Expressive Lives of Elders* (2018): 27–41, DOI: 10.2979/expressivelivesofelders.0.0.02

Dakota and Indiana, respectively (Geist 2017; Kay 2016a). Additionally, the media amplified the creative aging movement. Stories about "the road to superaging" (Barrett 2016), applied oral histories as tools for caregivers (Bahrampour 2016), and Glen Campbell's 2012 farewell tour caught my attention professionally and personally. Physicians diagnosed my father in 2007 with an early onset dementia that put him in a nursing home at sixty-one and killed him within two years; and a year ago, after two major surgeries, my mother moved into a long-term skilled care center where she tells me she is sometimes bored. They are two of many relatives and friends who entered, or may soon enter, the so-called golden years in the midst of new aging models.

As I participated in Missouri's Creative Aging Network and studied Geist's and Kay's work, I came back repeatedly to my anecdotal thinking and a question about folk artists and their lifelong engagement in traditional communities. What is it about traditional arts that seem to sustain their bearers? Based on years of research, Gene Cohen discovered a connection between artistic participation and elders' well-being; Troyd Geist developed projects that adapted traditional expressions for the benefits of residents in long-term care communities; and Jon Kay articulated the functions of memory objects for their makers. Most often, they (and I) worked with elders in retirement. These studies and projects brought us understanding about how the arts enhance wellness. For instance, when I first met old-time fiddler Cliff Bryan during a site visit in 2000, he was seventy-two years old and days away from the auction of his family's farm in rural Pomona, Missouri (population 511). Like many master artists we work with, Cliff's expressive life followed a trajectory—one where he was personally driven to learn a tradition as a child, eagerly sought out his elders for instruction, practiced diligently, and interacted socially. In much of adulthood, though, Cliff sidetracked often from his music and its social traditions to earn a living and raise his family. After the auction, Cliff and Sue, his wife, moved twelve miles away to the city of West Plains, where they lived in a sweet ranch house and hosted weekly music parties in their kitchen for seventeen years. Between 2000 and 2016, Cliff also taught six students in our statewide Traditional Arts Apprenticeship Program, passing a regional old-time fiddling style down to his younger students. From the first to the sixth apprenticeships, we noticed that with weekly (likely daily) fiddling, this established master artist continued to improve his artistry. By the seventh apprenticeship, his fiddling began to decline some due to age, but the apprenticeship was successful as he still recalled and shared a massive repertoire of tunes—with a little prompting. In large part, Cliff lived to fiddle; it brought him great joy, a joy that he knew up until his last days in March 2017.

I have known many other master artists whose traditions sustained and seemingly healed them. In her early seventies, German bobbin lace maker Christa Robbins of Dixon, Missouri, suffered a stroke, yet seemed to recover almost fully because she was so intent on making lace again. *Kloppelei*, something she learned as a little girl in East Germany, appeared to be her best therapy. While her penmanship grew wobbly, Christa made intricate, impeccable lace by juggling dozens of bobbins between both hands. African American storyteller Gladys Coggswell suffered a very debilitating stroke in 2005. I know from our conversations that she initially did not have much hope to recover fully or to ever gather and share stories again. With prodding from her family, apprentices, and presenters, storytelling again became a lure for Gladys, and she recovered her speech, her voice, and her determination. In addition to storytelling, she embarked on several documentation projects. Master dulcimer musician and luthier Don Graves of Lebanon, Missouri, once told my coworker Deborah Bailey how much his family tradition meant to him. This conversation was during his bout with colon cancer, just before a public performance on a warm June afternoon. Don told her, "I *live* for this" (emphasis added), fully signaling that despite being nauseous and weak that particular day from chemotherapy, he was determined to get up on stage. He intended to perform cherished tunes with his sister that their father passed down to them on instruments made by Don, his father, and great-grandfather. That was how he chose to live.

At eighty-four, Doris Frazier continues to direct choirs at Union Baptist Church in historic Westland Acres in the St. Louis metro area and to teach gospel piano to two exceptional teenage boys. Octogenarians H. K. Silvey, Alvie Dooms, and Gordon McCann strive to jam on Monday nights at the former McClurg General Store in southern Missouri. Their mileage varies. Alvie rarely misses a week as the group's rhythm guitarist, and I find myself gauging H. K. and Gordon's health by how often they appear in videos posted to the McClurg Jam's Facebook page each Tuesday morning. At age ninety-four, Kirkwood's Vesta Johnson fiddles every day, teaches fiddle camp every summer, and travels with her grandson and apprentice to play major festivals as far away as Washington and West Virginia. After Barranquilla, Colombia–to–St. Louis transplant Carmen Sofia Dence retired in 2015 from a career in radiology research, she increased her folkloric dance troupe's performances and founded a second dance troupe—one dedicated to older and wiser women like herself. Over almost two decades, I have quietly theorized that these artists' personal commitments to their traditional lives not only bring them joy but also help them to bear, and sometimes overcome, life's more stressful milestones and adversities. Through their traditions, they hope to live fully and not simply exist. Traditional arts serve as physical, occupational, and emotional therapies, as these artists embellish and polish their golden years in retirement, whether retirement is a few years or decades.

In this chapter, I want to focus on another artist who continues in his family's tradition and occupation. Eight years ago, because of a dire diagnosis and prognosis, he retired. While the diagnosis was accurate, thankfully, the progno-

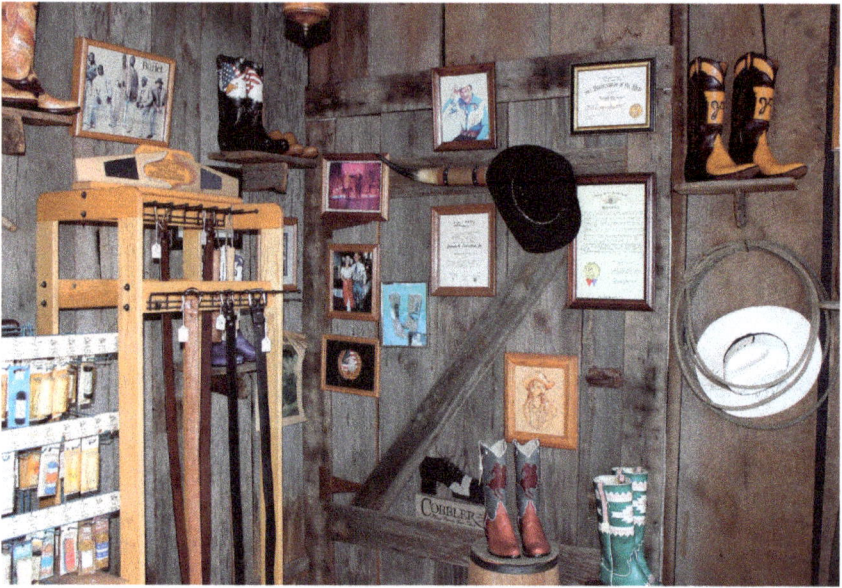

Fig. 1.1. The Patrickus family has adorned the showroom of JP's Boots with awards, procla-
mations, client photos, retail items, and several pairs of boots that highlight the bootmakers' skills. *Photograph by Lisa L. Higgins.*

sis was inaccurate, or, as I suspect, fifth-generation master western bootmaker
Joseph Patrickus Jr. beat the odds of that diagnosis, in part, due to a foundation
in his family legacy and his own artistic expressions. From 1978 until 2009, Joe
was the sole proprietor of JP's Custom Handmade Boots in Camdenton, Missouri. After Joe's retirement, his son Joseph Patrickus III took over running the
business, which is now on the cusp of its fortieth anniversary. Unlike the artists
described above, Joe pursued artistic expression within his primary occupation
in material culture, rather than beyond the workday or mostly in retirement. Joe
still lives to create, though. Retirement be damned; he is creating at the shop or
at home.

Many travelers might miss a small shop tucked in at the crossroads of Missouri Highway 54 and Highway 5 in the heart of Camdenton, a community with
a population just under 4,000 that is embraced by the southwest arms of the
manmade Lake of the Ozarks. Lake of the Ozarks is centrally located in Missouri
and a quick drive as well from bordering states. "The Lake," as Missourians call
it, is a wildly popular recreational and professional destination in central Missouri. The natural landscape—broad expanses of water and grand cliffs covered
in deciduous trees—is stunning in any season. JP's Custom Handmade Boots

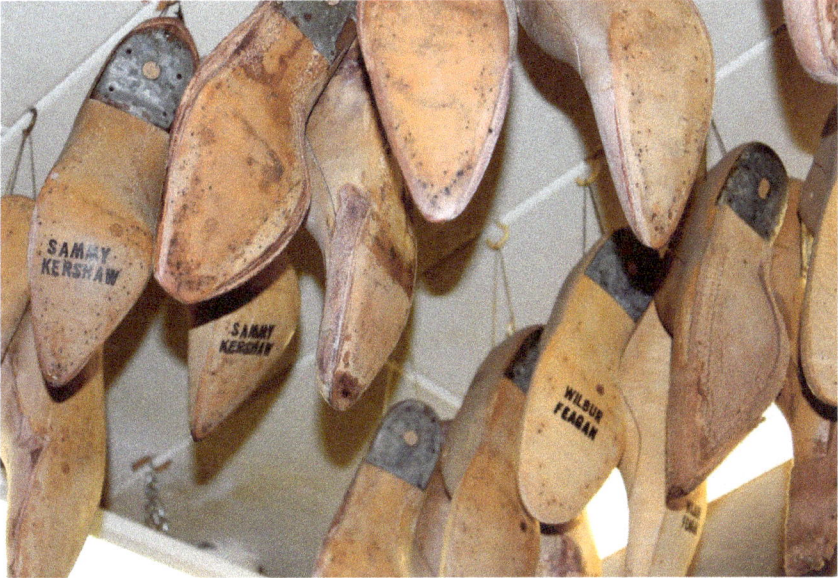

Fig. 1.2. Clients' boot lasts, often tagged with their names, hang from the ceiling of the shop. *Photograph by Lisa L. Higgins.*

sits at one end of a small arc of local businesses in vintage buildings, next door to a probation service agency and a land surveyor. A traveler waiting in heavy seasonal traffic for a red light to change to green might glance twice at the rustic wooden facade of JP's Boots, adorned with a large black, red, and white cutout of a western boot. One window is inscribed *Bootmaker* and the second *Shoe Repair*. Above the shake shingle awning, the proprietor has wood-burned the words *custom* and *handmade* onto two signs. JP's exterior would fit right in on a dusty street in the Old West. Stepping inside the swinging door, one faces a vintage counter, the boundary between customer service and workspaces. A small showroom sits to the right of the entrance, more accurately described as a self-curated exhibit rather than a retail space. On the other side of a thick braided rope, Patrickus displays several pairs of intricate, colorful, and quite stunning boots. Some boot tops are hand etched while others feature inlays depicting images ranging from the shop's logo on alligator and an American flag behind a bald eagle to a bucking horse and rider. Exotic skin belts hang from a display. Framed awards, client photos, and newspaper stories adorn the weathered wooden walls (fig. 1.1).

Ryan Habermeyer (2007, 10–11), a Missouri Folk Arts Program graduate assistant, wrote about his first impression walking into JP's Boots: "I'm admittedly mesmerized by an assortment of shoe 'lasts' dangling from the ceiling. 'Their placement is a practical decision,' Joe tells me. A way to create more space in a small shop, but its old-west charm is aesthetically seductive. Like ghosts of shoes previously created—and those not yet created. These incredibly dense, carved blocks of Canadian maple . . . shaped into an abstract concept of a foot, are the most fundamental objects in the cordwainer's trade. The last is the soul of the shoe." Lasts are the soul of the shoe and have been the soul of JP's Boots (fig. 1.2).

For baby boomers and older millennials, movie heroes, such as Roy Rogers, and television stars, such as the Lone Ranger, made western boots highly desirable for youngsters in the 1950s. Urban cowboys later bloomed in the 1980s, and, more recently, rural brides, grooms, and wedding parties sporting boots are de rigueur. In addition to having pop culture appeal, contemporary boot production, as geographer Chris Gibson has noted, is both "place and path dependent," such as with western boot production in El Paso, Texas. There, proximity to cultural traditions and a skilled migrant pool of makers created a production boomtown where companies such as Cowtown Boots, Lucchese, and Justin Boots relocated and thrived (Gibson 2016, 73). So, we may ask, how does a solo western bootmaker find his home in the heart of the Missouri Ozarks, in the midst of lake culture and business conference centers? Most people in the United States today do not associate Missouri with the Old (or New) West, with cowboys, or even country western musicians. Missouri, though, is the birthplace of the ornately suited and booted Porter Wagoner, bluegrass virtuoso Rhonda Vincent, and the folk hero/cold-blooded killer Jesse James. Missouri is the "Gateway to the West," marked by that futuristic arch hovering over the Mississippi River. Missouri, too, is home to Branson's country music theaters and frontier-themed Silver Dollar City amusement park. Even *Modern Family* sitcom character Cam Tucker knows that Missouri has "a very vibrant cowboy poetry scene." Perhaps, then, it is not surprising that our quasi-western state, earned through folklore and fakelore, claims a handful of custom western boot–making shops, including JP's, which was established in 1978.

JP is Joseph Patrickus Jr. (or "the second," as he prefers). One might think a former electronics engineer born and raised in the heart of urban Chicago is an unexpected master western bootmaker in Missouri or to the west. Indeed, Joe spent a decade or so in his first career, successfully working at companies such as General Telephone & Electronics Laboratories and Motorola. In the mid-1970s, he "ditched his suit," and his new path brought Joe to a new place in rural Missouri with Marcella, his beloved wife, and their growing family. A "maker," then and now, Joe and his eldest son, Joey (then fourteen), first set to constructing the family's finely crafted and spacious two-story log home. Joe used his engineering experience to draw up blueprints, and they harvested much of the raw materials from their rural property near the unincorporated community of Macks Creek,

Missouri, in Camden County. Around this time, Joe also decided to go into the "family trade" for his second career. He had learned the basics alongside his dad as a boy, and two uncles still worked in the business:

> They were the last ones in the trade. My grandfather had passed away. Even my own father worked, when [he and my mother] first got married, for my grandfather in Iowa at his shops. And my two uncles, well, [they] actually worked for my grandfather before World War II. In World War II . . . they were put in on the second wave of the Normandy invasion . . . and they ended up repairing all the military boots for the Australians, and the French, and stuff like that. And after World War II, they moved to Peoria, Illinois, in 1949. And [then] they moved out to Sacramento, and they were the last ones in the trade because all the older people had passed away. Of course, they always wanted me to go into the trade. (Joseph F. Patrickus, Jr., interview with author, February 22, 2017)

As Joe and Joey were building the family home, Joe researched the family business, and an opportunity appeared to buy out the key tools of a cobbler's shop in Macks Creek. Joe picked up the phone and called his uncle Aldie, the World War II veteran now living in California:

> Told my uncle this is what I want to do. And he said, "Nah," and I was gonna buy some equipment, and he said, "No, stay with what you're doing!" Whatever, and I said, "No, this is what I'm doing. Made up my mind."
> So I called him the next day, and I said, "I bought this stuff." And he said, "OK, I'm on the bus; I'll be on my way out." And so he came out, and we spent every bit of sixteen, eighteen hours a day just going through everything. And I can't even tell you how long he was here, but it was a long time. Went through all the basics, all the information that was needed. (Joseph F. Patrickus, Jr., interview with author, February 22, 2017)

After that intensive apprenticeship with Uncle Aldie, Joe, now the fifth generation in the business, opened his first shop in Macks Creek. Six months later, he outgrew that shop and opened JP's Boot—the little shop on Camdenton's US Highway 54. Joe outfitted his business with the used equipment that sparked Uncle Aldie's long bus ride. A few years later, Joe purchased more equipment from the estate of Mac McDaniels in St. Louis, including an 1898 lathe that shaped the foundation of the boots—and Joe's business (fig. 1.3).

Another folklorist once told me in an offhand way, "Oh, bootmakers are a dime a dozen." They are not, and Joe is not. With the traditional knowledge passed down from four generations, Joe Patrickus has been a unique bootmaker. Additionally, he spent several hours observing and learning from Mac McDaniels in St. Louis, as he and his staff fashioned lasts on the lathe that Joe later acquired. Joe turned his formal training in design, his traditional training from Uncle Aldie, and his informal training with McDaniels into high-quality work,

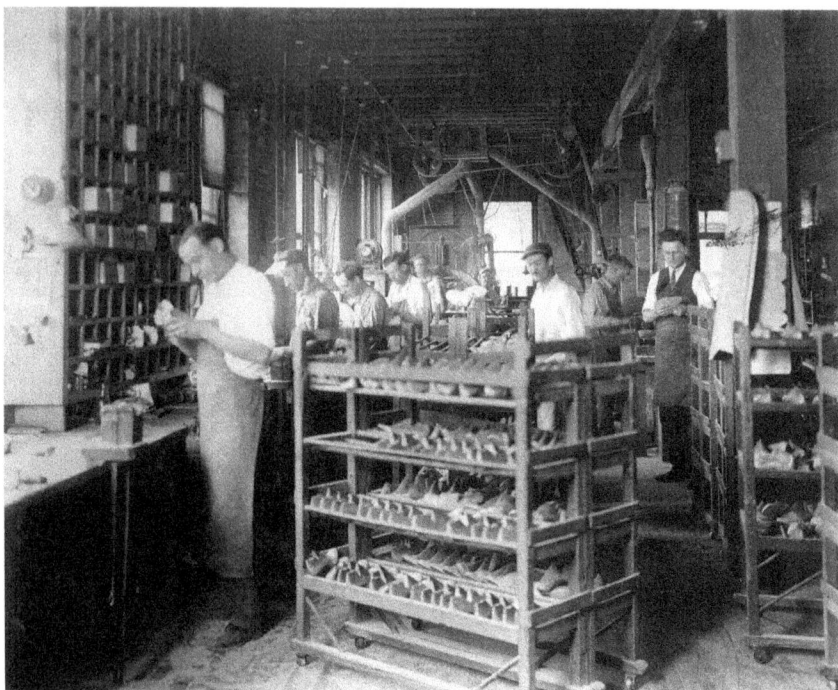

Fig. 1.3. Joe Patrickus keeps this historic photograph of Mac MacDaniels's St. Louis last making business in a frame on the wall of JP's Boots. *Courtesy of Joseph F. Patrickus II.*

both subtle and elaborate. For many decades, Joe also made custom lasts—wooden forms turned out from his large stock of Canadian hard maple. Lasts make all the difference in the world for a custom fit, for adapting to hammer toes or bunions, flat feet or high arches, and other individual distinctions. Rather than amending prefab plastic forms like many bootmakers and cobblers, Joe turned custom lasts for his clients. Then, in the evenings in those earlier years, Joe would turn lasts for other shops to make ends meet, to support his family, and to grow his business, which he did with endless hours, fine craft, and word-of-mouth advertising.

In more than thirty years as the sole proprietor of JP's Boots, Joe fashioned custom works of art for hundreds of well-heeled and everyday clients, including actor/director/governor Arnold Schwarzenegger; Egyptian business magnate Mohamed Al-Fayed; country music artist Sammy Kershaw; Springfield, Missouri, dairy expert Wilbur Feagan; and my friend Kitty Rogers, a family therapist in mid-Missouri. Tyler Beard, author and western boot expert, highlighted

Joe's artistry in 2006 by including him as one of only twenty-seven artists in the popular *Art of the Boot* (Beard and Arndt 1999). Joe also earned recognition and esteem as he exhibited boots at the (former) Roy Rogers Museum in Branson, Missouri, and the Buffalo Bill Museum in Golden, Colorado. In 2003, the George H. W. Bush Library and Museum in College Station, Texas, awarded Joseph Patrickus Jr. the Director's Choice Award at the 2003 *Legends of the West* exhibition.

In addition to his prolific recognition with private clients, at trade shows, and in public exhibitions, Joe taught in Missouri's Traditional Arts Apprenticeship program five times from 1997 to 2007. He taught a son, a daughter, and two friends. In 2006, Joe discovered that I collect children's cowboy boots for decorative display, and he pointed me to the magnificent eye candy that photographer Jim Arndt provided to illustrate Beard's books. On that day, I mentally added a pair of custom JP's boots to my bucket list. At that time, Joe was a young and vibrant sixty-year-old, and he had spent decades already mastering and making what he calls with pride "functional art." To comprehend the extent of his artistic trade, it has been helpful for me to visit him at the shop over the years. Once, I stopped by JP's Boots, and Joe sat at a drafting table in the back of the shop sketching representational images of fluffy cotton bolls and fat catfish (iconic symbols in southeastern Missouri). He was mocking up the design for a homesick Missouri attorney working as a fund-raiser and lobbyist in Washington, DC.

For this client and hundreds of others, Joe created what Jon Kay (2016a, 3) calls "memory objects," or "material forms of life stories." Unlike woodcarver Bob Taylor, rug hooker Marian Sykes, and walking cane carver John Schoolman, the featured artists in Kay's book *Folk Art and Aging*, Joe Patrickus rarely creates his own memory objects. He has not mapped his personal "life review" onto his own boots but can trace his artistic "life review" in dozens of ledgers where clients' feet are outlined in pencil, in manila file folders that hold notes and designs traced onto paper, and in images stored on a stack of dusty computer discs. Joe can even look up at the ceiling of his shop, where lasts hang and recall the clients and their special orders. He is a storyteller, an interpreter, an ethnographer, a seer who interprets other peoples' stories in wood, leathers, pegs, and threads. Examples of these memory objects span a wide range from subtle to elaborate.

For my friend Kitty Rogers, Joe embroidered a simple rendition of her tattoo, a snake with a flower for its head, onto each outer front upper. She chose red French calfskin boots in 2002, she says, to match her red Chevy truck. She wrote that

> His shop felt like home. Or a museum. So comfortable, like Joe. He listed off the celebrities he made boots for, not boastingly, so much as matter of factly. His boots were beautiful. He explained the process in detail, let me touch the leather. We talked at length about what I wanted. I put a deposit down and came back a few months later to pick them up. They were beautiful. Fit like a

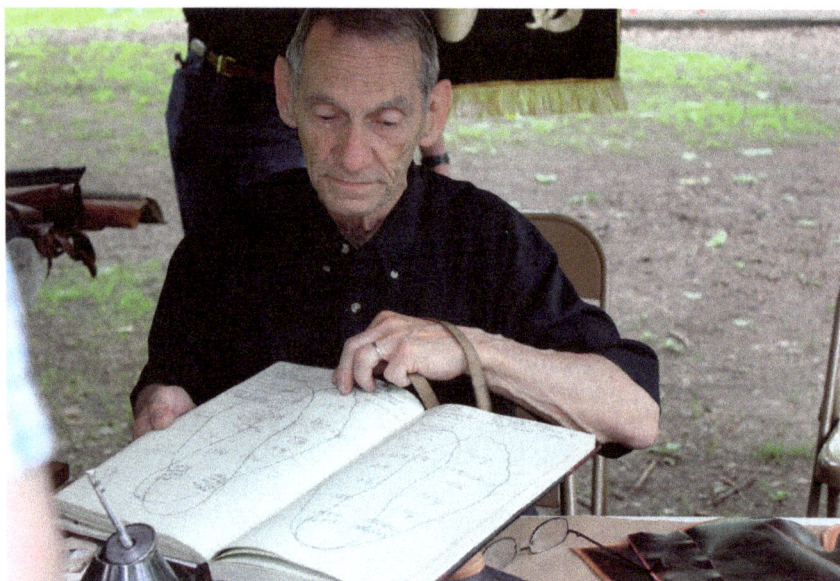

Fig. 1.4. Joe Patrickus explains to a festival visitor how he records a client's measurements in a ledger. *Photograph by Heather Rhodes Johnson for the Missouri Folk Arts Program.*

glove. Because they were red, they attracted a lot of attention. I loved telling people they were HANDMADE. How often do we get to see handmade boots?

They are still beautiful, a little worn, like my feet. Sometimes, I use them as a vase, so I can look at them, the most expensive pair of boots I've ever owned. But they're art. Joe is the artist. (Kitty Rogers, letter to author, August 25, 2017)

Fifteen years later, Kitty Rogers is still enamored with her boots, with the memory inscribed on leather, the memory of the consultation with the artist, and the muscle memories of wearing and displaying her boots. Joe Patrickus customized a work of art that evokes one vignette in Kitty's life, attaining a check mark on her personal bucket list.

Roy Rogers commissioned Joe to build an elaborately adorned reproduction of the singing cowboy's signature Double-Eagles, a nod to the late Texas bootmaker Charlie Garrison's original design. That signed and numbered boot series was in honor of Roy and Dale Evans's fiftieth wedding anniversary in 1997, embellished with diamonds to signify their major milestone. For Arnold Schwarzenegger's fifty-fifth birthday, Joe rendered images from the movie *Terminator 3* onto full alligator boot tops: a Humvee, the new T-X model terminator, and a director's clapboard are inlayed. Joe consulted on that pair from start to finish by

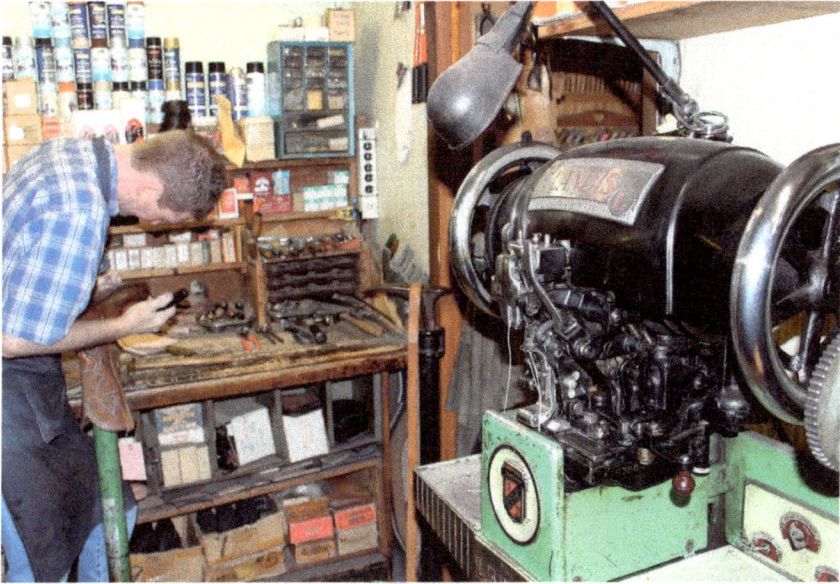

Fig. 1.5. Joseph F. Patrickus III replaces a boot's sole in the shop's workroom. He works daily with hand tools and vintage machines like the outsole stitcher in the foreground. *Photograph by Lisa L. Higgins.*

phone with the actor's wife and best friend, as a surprise birthday gift. In each of these examples, and so many others, Joe Patrickus has rendered memories into "material legacies" (Kay 2016b, 144). Joe works with his clients to honor their milestones, allude to bygone days, and capture moments in popular culture.

Before translating his clients' wishes into designs, Joe takes meticulous measurements of the client's feet, insteps, ankles, and calves (both sides, as no one is symmetrical). He records all in a ledger (fig. 1.4). As the consultation deepens, Joe gathers the client's story, motifs, and preferences. He consults about leathers, inlays, stitches, "toe flowers and wrinkles," pulls (or "mule ears"), heels, caps, and collars. Where the client provides input and inspiration, Joe guides decisions about design, materials, color schemes, and finishes. This traditional artist employs many techniques; he sketches, designs, etches, carves, sews, chisels, embroiders, pieces, and inlays. He sometimes bejewels. Joe also works on many canvases (tracing paper, wood, and leathers) to produce one work of art—or more accurately, a pair. In his first steps of construction, with measurements recorded and designs sketched, Joe turns lasts—precise wooden forms turned on the 1898 lathe—onto which he shapes the boots' vamps. As boot enthusiast Jennifer June (2007, 278) points out in *Cowboy Boots: The Art & Sole*, "the last captures . . . boots interior space, incorporating both the foot width and diameter, and also the toe shape and heel height." The lasts are the boots' physical foundation. The boot-maker shapes the damp leather of the vamp over the last, and when it dries, the maker removes the last, leaving negative space for the client's foot. After serving their fundamental role, JP's lasts are stored on hooks in the shop's ceiling—for a second or third pair of boots in the future.

Eight years ago, Joe retired from JP's Boots, and Joseph Patrickus III (JP3) took over as proprietor, running all day-to-day operations (fig. 1.5). Like his dad, Joey had learned the family trade in his youth. Like his dad, Joey also chose a different career path first. Joe chose electronics, and Joey chose law enforcement. For Joey's second career, together father and son adapted the shop for its next era. Among other choices, they downsized square footage and sold the 1898 lathe. When I learned that the lathe was for sale, I worried. I had come to think of the lathe as JP's foundation. At this time, Joe had not shared his diagnosis with me, and I had not been in contact as regularly after his last apprenticeship. He would call me unexpectedly on occasion, once to ask if I knew a yarn spinner. I was first surprised, then amused, as Joe explained that he wondered if he could repurpose his Great Pyrenees dog's hair into yarn. Always thinking creatively! In December 2014, Joe and Marcella visited the office of the Missouri Folk Arts Program before their appointment at the veterans' hospital in Columbia. They arrived as animated and vibrant as ever, although Joe breathed a little harder than usual and towed a portable oxygen tank. He explained to us, in a roundabout way, that he was not well, but he also said that as long as he was around, he was always up to help the Missouri Folk Arts Program in any way. The latter statement, by the way, was not a new refrain. Six months later, we took him up on that offer. Joe and Joey were featured demonstrators at a mini-festival in southwest Missouri for the apprenticeship program's thirtieth anniversary. They drove more than two hours one way and, of course, arrived early for setup. They greeted park visitors throughout the day, showing off exotic leathers, boots in progress, and three finished pairs from the showroom. An exhausting day for everyone, and Joe smiled through the whole thing. He was living for it.

In 2016, I initiated a conversation with Joe; I wanted to write about a traditional craftsperson and aging, and I had always wanted to interview him, to learn more about his art, and to hear the stories behind the stories he transcribed on his clients' boots. Joe agreed, and we met twice for face-to-face interviews—at his home in February 2017 and at the shop in May 2017. We also talked on the telephone and exchanged e-mails. It was in February that Joe defined his concept of a "basket list," which he had mentioned on the phone when we arranged the interview. By this time, almost everyone has heard of a bucket list—life goals to check off before we are incapable. As Joe continues to live his customized life with a chronic illness, he has found a metaphor for the improvisations he must make when a goal becomes unattainable: "Yeah, a basket instead of a bucket because my basket doesn't hold everything. Sometimes things slip through." I acknowledged, and Joe agreed, that making boots was still a top priority; boot making does not slip out of the basket. He has not retired fully; he is at the shop every morning when health permits (and sometimes even when it does not). Joe was, and still is, a full-time craftsman; only the definition of "full time" has been revised, not the definition of "craftsman." Speaking in present tense in 2017, he told me that for so many, boot making is a side business or a profitable hobby: "There's maybe less than a dozen of us that do it professionally. That's our way of life." Joe has a love for the work, and Joey still requests that his dad collaborate often. Joe jokes that he comes in regularly to "pick up his paycheck." He also notes that his son never hesitates to call or nudge, request input, or ask for help with a backlog. Joey reminds Joe to stay artistically engaged, and the elder is determined to be in the shop. As he remarked on the phone in September 2017, "I don't give up in here; I just don't come in six days a week."

It seems the timing, at least, of Joe's so-called retirement was perfect. First, Joey retired from law enforcement. He was ready to return to the shop and make boots full time. Then, Joe acknowledges:

> It was a health decision. I'm a very stubborn person. When somebody says I got six months to two years, I'm there to prove that wrong. But for health reasons, yeah, I had to cut back my time. I thought it was time for Joey to take the reins and control of things. Eventually, it was going to be his. And at sixty-two, it was the time to do it. And I didn't give up on it. It was time to make that transition, and so he could take full responsibility, and I could sit back and watch from the grandstand. (Joseph F. Patrickus, Jr., interview with author, February 22, 2017)

Joe Patrickus does not watch from the grandstand. Some days, he must tweak his path and his place, but he rarely quits. He drives his middle son, Bill, to work twenty minutes into Camdenton many days and heads to work over at JP's. And Joe has that basket list. Possibly, spinning Great Pyrenees yarn fell out of the basket, but last May, he fashioned an inexpensive solar heater for his well house from upcycled aluminum soda cans and plate glass from his Mennonite neighbors. Now that the weather has turned cooler, he reports that the project is a success and plans to build three more to use at JP's Boots. Joe also recently turned his attention to the business's website, which he and his daughter Kate built years ago, finding someone to help him with updates. He and his daughter Jennifer, who lives next door on the homestead, are deeply involved in capturing the family genealogy; they have happened upon a ship manifest that Joe believes may indicate that the boot-making tradition goes back more than six generations. In our February 2017 conversation, he said that Joey tells him "you need to record some of this, Dad." Joey's request and my interest dovetailed there, and I am working to help record some of those stories. In May, I visited Joe at the shop, and he scrolled through some boot designs and photos saved to discs. At the Missouri Folk Arts Program, our student workers have transcribed the first two interviews, and we will pair Joe's stories with the images that I snapped in JP's office. We have not set a time yet, but I plan to visit again to record more stories and images. I have made it a project that is on my bucket list, and I hope it stays in Joe's basket list for a long while.

My relationship with Joe Patrickus, as an artist and a friend, is not unique in the field of public folklore. So many of us have developed these relationships of wonder and mutual admiration with traditional artists. I hesitate to posit any universal truths based on anecdotes, observations, or even my conversations with Joe. My own professional experiences easily reveal stories that are the exceptions; too many artists, with strong wills to live and to express themselves creatively, did not eclipse fate. Over the last twelve months, we at the Missouri Folk Arts Program, for instance, have bid farewell to too many. From the thirty-nine-year-old to the eighty-nine-year-old, each had much to live for and so much more to learn and to share. In the midst of his personal, professional, and somatic knowledge that the only certainties are uncertainties, Joe Patrickus, his stories, and his metaphors remind me to work hard, follow dreams, share stories, and always remain adaptable. The wooden last of Canadian hard maple is a boot's fixed foundation, yet Joe knows that he can amend it, as clients' feet and bodies change. Even JP's finished works of art can be periodically repaired, resoled, repolished, shored up, and rejuvenated. Similarly, his basket is a vessel, and a metaphor, that holds objects and goals, but the basket is not a bucket. As Joe pointed out, his "basket" is small and porous—it holds less, and some goals might seep or fall out depending on the day and the circumstances. These material objects, then, are Joe's metaphors that may resonate with others, as they do for me both personally and professionally. In addition to taking away a profound understanding of his customized "functional art," I also have deeper glimpses of Joe's accomplishments, his struggles, and his wisdom that cannot help but inform how I work and how I live.

LISA L. HIGGINS is Director of the Missouri Folk Arts Program, a Missouri Arts Council partner based at the Museum of Art and Archaeology at the University of Missouri.

## Works Cited

Bahrampour, Tara. 2016. "This Former Journalist Helps Caregivers Get to Know Who Their Patients Once Were, before Dementia Took Hold." *Washington Post*, December 15.

Barrett, Lisa Feldman. 2016. "How to Become a 'Superager.'" *New York Times*, December 31.

Beard, Tyler, and Arndt, Jim. 1999. *The Art of the Boot*. Layton, UT: Gibbs Smith.

Cohen, Gene D., Susan Perlstein, Jeff Chapline, Jeanne Kelly, Kimberly M. Firth, and Samuel Simmens. 2006. "The Impact of Professionally Conducted Cultural Programs on the Physical Health, Mental Health, and Social Functioning of Older Adults." *The Gerontologist* 46: 726–34.

Geist, Troyd A. 2017. *Sundogs and Sunflowers: An Art for Life Program Guide for Creative Aging, Health, and Wellness*. Bismarck: North Dakota Council on the Arts.

Gibson, Chris. 2016. "Material Inheritances: How Place, Materiality, and Labor Process Underpin the Path-Dependent Evolution of Contemporary Craft Production." *Economic Geography* 92 (1): 60–88.

Habermeyer, Ryan. 2007. "The Magic of Bootmaking." *Museum Magazine* 71: 10–11.

June, Jennifer. 2007. *Cowboy Boots: The Art and Sole*. New York: Universe Publishing.

Kay, Jon. 2016a. *Folk Art and Aging: Life-Story Objects and Their Makers*. Bloomington: Indiana University Press.

———. 2016b. "Life Story Objects: Folk Art and Aging in Indiana." In *Material Vernaculars: Objects, Images, and Their Social Worlds*, edited by Jason Baird Jackson, 143–59. Bloomington: Indiana University Press.

# 2    Aging with Grace and Power

## A Puerto Rican Healer's Story

### Selina Morales

L ET ME INTRODUCE you to a woman who works as a traditional healer. Her stories will help reveal how attention to the roles of traditional arts and community-embedded cultural practices in one's life can widen our understanding of the process of aging. In this case, I tell a story of a woman who stays connected to her community through her use of traditional healing arts. The story focuses on ways that storytelling about these healing practices has helped to build power, contributing to her ability to continue to labor for others as she approached the age of ninety. I ask, what role does her ongoing healing practice have in maintaining her own well-being? How does this community-centered work heal the healer?

I have had the special opportunity to learn from this healer for nearly four decades. As I have aged, her stories have changed, offering me age-appropriate touchstones as well as different ways of understanding her choices. Like many before me, I have chosen to write a personal account of my experiences as a listener and as an actor in the production of stories I've shared here (see Kirshenblatt and Kirshenblatt-Gimlett 2007; Myerhoff 1978; Hurston 1935; McCarthy Brown 2001; Trinh 1989). In this chapter, I sift through eighteen years of recordings of fluid conversations about a life as a healer, giving special attention to the ways that Jerusalén Morales tells stories about her power and her grace and to the ways that community healing work combats the loneness, isolation, and uselessness that might have disrupted her vital role as a community healthcare worker:

> I have a special grace; people sit down to talk to me for hours. They tell me, "You know what you are doing is special; not everybody can do what you are

*The Expressive Lives of Elders* (2018): 42–54, DOI: 10.2979/expressivelivesofelders.0.0.03

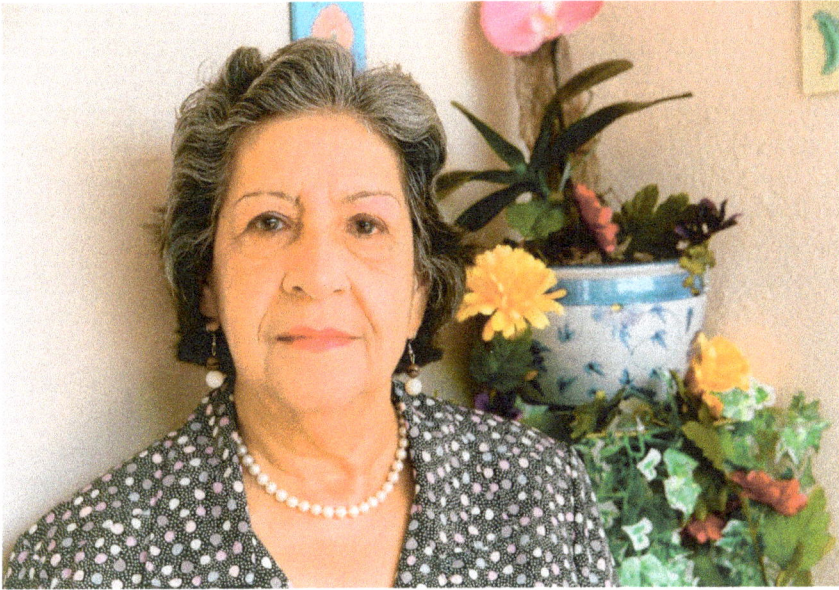

Fig. 2.1. Jerusalén Morales at her home in Naranjito, Puerto Rico. *Photograph by Selina Morales, 2006.*

doing." Not everybody can do the things I do. . . . You don't have to be an *espiritista* [healer], but a person that when you speak or talk, you enter [another] person's heart. Like if you are a singer, when you sing a song, you move the audience. . . . When you cure a wound, it hurts; but after a while, it feels much better. The same thing [happens] when you talk to a person, maybe the person cries or maybe they feel mad at you; but after that moment, you [change] that person. And that is the grace of a healer; a spirit goes through the hands of the healer to make a moment so beautiful, like when you light a match, you light that person's life. That is how you know you have the power to heal. . . . You have to be humble, accept it with dignity and grace. (Jerusalén Morales, age seventy-two)

My grandmother, Jerusalén Morales (fig. 2.1), is a Puerto Rican *espiritista* healer.[1] She communicates with metaphysical beings, with spirits, in order to offer advice to her community. She also concocts remedies to cure a range of ailments from stomachache to heartache. Her own proficiency as a healer is measured by her facility with the aesthetic codes connected to *espiritismo*/spiritism. For more than fifty years, her communities (Latinos in the Bronx, Puerto Rico, Orlando, and people across the world via telephone) have relied on her wisdom and her proven connection to the spirit world as they move through their daily lives. Her critical community work keeps our heartaches short, puts our planes on course, cures whatever ails us, and even (and often) saves our lives through a practiced mixture of listening, advice giving, spirit channeling, and medicine making.

Over her lifetime as a worker, she has moved from the Bronx, New York, to rural Puerto Rico to St. Cloud, Florida. The manner of delivering of her services has shifted over her lifelong career. And over this time, she has had opportunities to demonstrate her expertise and proficiency as a healer as she has risen to environmental challenges (urban, rural, and suburban), always proving that she has the power and grace needed to cure her community.[2] These gifts and her work as a healer have had an immense impact on her own well-being as she ages and continues the hard labor of taking care of her community. Over my life, she has taught me how to do her healing work, including lessons in character, morality, self-reliance, trust, and faith. The stories she has shared with me have served as markers of her accomplishments. They also highlight her power over authority figures or her ways of subverting them and her particular phenomenal ability to heal others, her grace.

## A Cooking Lesson

It is 2001. Jerusalén and I are rolling *sorullitos de maíz* (fried corn sticks) at her kitchen table in Naranjito, Puerto Rico. The cornmeal is sticking to my fingers, but it glides easily on her hands as she expertly crafts uniform cigars with our salty-sweet yellow *masa*. We've made nearly a hundred, and I can easily tell hers from mine. The lard is heating in a black cast-iron pan. The thick, hot air smells rich and sweet. My grandmother picks up a small ball of dough and rolls it through her fingers:

> Selina, when I was younger, I got big problems in my life. One day, I became completely blind; I could not see my children, I could not see the stairs. So I started crying and I heard a voice that told me, "Don't cry. I am going to give you a third eye. You are going to see more than what you see now. Gather your children and go to the hospital. No operation has to be done on your eye. You just go there, and they are going to put some medicine on your eyes that smells like flowers, and when you've got that smell in your nose, you know you will be released of this blindness."
>
> So, I gathered my children, your father and all my children, and I went to the hospital. The doctor didn't find nothing wrong with my eyes. He said, "I don't know, you've got like a veil that won't let you see. So we are going to try a medicine that will smell like roses." When they put the medicine on my eyes, I smelled the roses. He said, "Wait here ten minutes because after this exam, we are going to make you another exam and if this doesn't work, then we have to do something else to you." So it passed ten minutes, and the doctor passed me the hands [in front of my eyes] and I did see the finger of the doctor. And he

said, "Can you see my finger?" I said, "Yes, I can see." So I stand up from the table and went home.

*Fijate bien*, Selina, pay attention. Oshun was the one who told me that, specifically Oshun, "Your third eye is going to open your life." From that day on, I start seeing things and I start saying it and the same way I said it, they come out. I was not listening before I received my telepathy—after I got my [third] eye open, I start listening to them talking to me. I was not scared at all; I liked it. It was like I was playing with someone that nobody sees but me and I was talking with someone that no one knows. Sometimes I caught myself talking alone, but I was answering questions that they ask me and I learned from there. From my own experience.[3] (Jerusalén Morales, age seventy-one)

This is the story Jerusalén shares when asked how she became a medium, but there had been earlier evidence. She was born Ramona Diaz in 1930 in San Juan, Puerto Rico, to Lorenzo and Juana Diaz. From her mother, she inherited the miraculous ability to communicate with the metaphysical. Jerusalén doesn't remember her mother, but she knows that they are connected through their shared dedication to community spirit work. Some family stories tell us that Juana knew her daughter Ramona was gifted with the power to heal others and changed her name to the more distinctive Jerusalén. Other family stories explain that Abuela Juana was so powerful that she prophesized her own death. On La Noche de San Juan, June 25, 1935, after baptizing herself in the sea, Abuela Juana went to sleep.[4] When she awoke from a night of active dreams, she knew that within a year, she would contract tuberculosis and leave behind her husband and two young daughters.

When Jerusalén discovered that she had psychic powers, she was a young mother living in the Bronx. She put her powers to use to both make a living and to heal people who, for economic, linguistic, and/or cultural reasons, lacked basic access to or faith in Western healthcare systems. Taking on this subversive public leadership role in her communities has been a point of pride throughout her life. Her healing stories have provided evidence of her power as she often recounts how male doctors, policemen, and other authority figures have been amazed (and often confounded) by her natural ability to work miracles.

## Brewing Tea

It is 2002, Jerusalén is seventy-two years old. After raising a family in the Bronx, she returned to Puerto Rico to live on a farm just outside the rural mountain town of Naranjito. I pop out of my bedroom to kiss my grandmother on the cheek and say good-night. She called from the kitchen, "I'm making *tila*." She has always been a night owl. I find her adding a teaspoon of sugar to a small saucepan of linden flower tea. She turns the sugar over and over as she explains, "This is to get my nerves to calm down. You can also do this with *naraja agria* [sour orange], the leaves." She pours the hot tea into two Corningware teacups. "This is delicious," she declares as she passes me two saucers and directs me to the dining table with her chin. "Sit down, Selina. I have to tell you." She pushes the tea toward me as we sit. For the past month, we've been recording stories about her early work as a healer in New York City, so my video camera is already poised for this session. I pressed the Record button, and she starts. "Selina, when the girl was born, she had a big, big, head. I mean big. And she had a little tiny body, like a fish. Her parents didn't know what to do. They went to see three different doctors." My grandmother holds her beautifully manicured hands in the air, thumb and pinkie touch and her long, cinnamon-colored fingers emphasize her point. Three doctors, no cure:

> The doctors didn't know what to do. Then the family came to see me at my *botánica.*[5] I took a look at the girl, and I knew. I went to the store and bought a coconut, the kind full of water, and I opened two of the eyes with a knife. I turned the coconut upside down and let the water drain out. I told the family to take the girl and go home, that the next day, they will see that her head would become small, and she would be a normal girl. I light a candle. Well, when the water drained out of that coconut, the girl was completely cured. Selina, the doctors couldn't believe it. When the girl went in for her next appointment, she was a normal girl. The doctor said, "How can this be? I want to meet this lady who cured this little girl." The doctors came to meet me, and they told me, "You have powers that we don't have. How can you do this?"
> My grandmother gives me a sly smile. "And the girl lived a long life."

She presents this story, and others like it, as evidence of her victories over a system that, throughout history, excludes her worldview from its canon. In her healing stories, she always confounds the presumed "know-it-all" and saves her people using the wisdom given to her by the spirits (that only she can hear and see). In these heroic tales, she gets invited to give lectures, teach classes, and otherwise share her knowledge with astonished healthcare professionals.

## Caring for Community

Success stories, like the one above, and the dozens of others I have recorded since 2001, serve as a way for Jerusalén to claim her life story, name her accomplishments, and to assert her status as a community-accredited healthcare provider. These stories are also ways that Jerusalén educates me. Early life lessons about resiliency, resourcefulness, and about locating power and trust within oneself have been valuable anchors for me, a woman of color growing up in the United States.

I was raised in a *botánica* in the South Bronx, surrounded by ritual objects of the Caribbean. I spent my childhood organizing decorated glass seven-day candles on shelves, filling jars with fragrant myrrh and herbs, and stocking pale pink rosaries. As the proprietor of the shop, Jerusalén offered her spiritual services to the large Caribbean community of the South Bronx. While she did her spirit work, she simultaneously cared for my brothers, my cousins, and me. As young people, we observed our grandmother working for her community, curing a range of ailments from seriously sick children to people who just wanted to change their luck. Her *botánica*, Jardines de Jerusalén, was open from 1985 to 1991.

Jerusalén explains, "A *botánica* is a pharmacy for the soul. . . . It is a place where people go to deal with their inner being, to seek remedies that will heal their spirits." *Botánicas* are stores that sell ritual merchandise necessary for practicing a variety of traditional Latin American belief systems. From love potions, lucky pennies, and statues of Catholic saints to fresh herbs and spiritual consultations, the *botánica* offers an alternative health resource to its community. Jerusalén's command of the paraphernalia in her *botánica*, her knowledge of dried herbs, artificially dyed potions, and clay statues made her, as proprietor, an important figure in her community.

At the center of a *botánica* are strong faith-based relationships. Whether between family, friends, or strangers; gods, spirits, ancestors, or nature; and the self, these relationships are nourished and encouraged through the products sold in the store. Jerusalén tells me that out of all the *botánicas* in the South Bronx, her clients/neighbors/friends chose to shop at Jardines de Jerusalén because they believed in her grace, in her ability to mediate between people and the spirit world.

The objects she sold were transformational. Her shop was a center of health and wellness in the low-income, largely immigrant neighborhood of the South Bronx. She sold aerosol cans whose scent brought luck, love, or money or could chase away evil. She sold fluorescent potions, religious amulets, fragrant oils, and rock incense. Also, she sold many objects that seemed mundane, everyday objects such as plants. It was her grace, the powers she imbued in pennies, for example, that turned them into extraordinary things: into lucky pennies.

## Making a Bath

It is 2006, two weeks before my wedding, and I am visiting with my grandparents on their farm in Naranjito. I am visiting to mark this major transition in my life, perhaps to glean some last wisdom before I approach a rite of passage, and, of course, we have work to do.

It has been raining for two days, and the clouds have finally passed. The ceramic dish we have left on the patio wall is now full of collected rainwater. Jerusalén calls me from the covered veranda as she picks up a broom and swiftly clears rainwater from the terra-cotta tiles. "Selina, pick some *mira-mi-linda* from

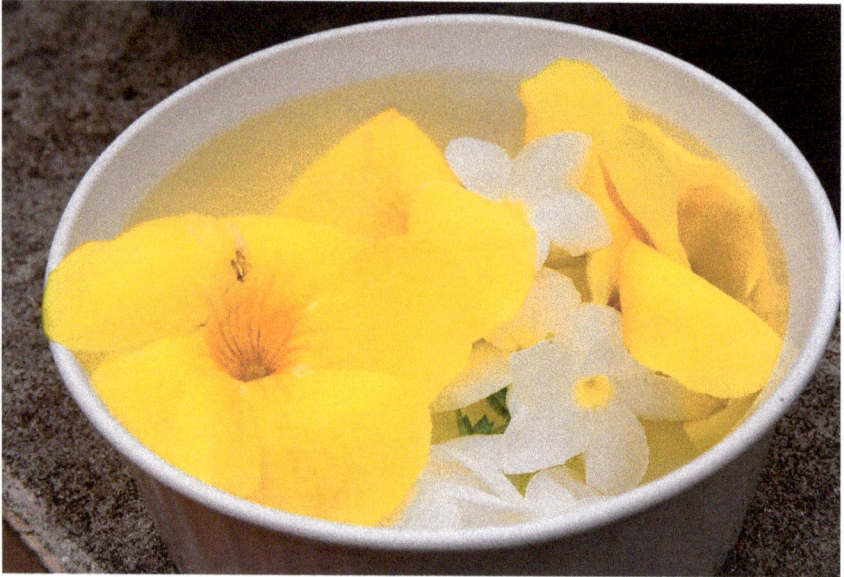

Fig. 2.2. Flowers gathered for a baño in Naranjito, Puerto Rico. *Photograph by Selina Morales, 2006.*

the yard, and bring some *canarios*, too." We are making a *baño* (literally, bath) for my brother, Ariel (fig. 2.2).

On her patio, Jerusalén has a small sour orange plant (the flowers and leaves of which are potent remedies for all kinds of sickness) and a large bird of paradise plant. She collects a few sour orange leaves and two buds from the bird of paradise. All of these plant parts are placed into the vessel with our collected rainwater and left in the hot Caribbean sun for an entire day. Jerusalén explains that the water soaks up the energy of the sun, activating the plants. The tonic will be potent.

After the sun energizes the mixture, Jerusalén recites quiet prayers, and she uses her hands to transfer her grace into the bath (fig. 2.3).[6] Next, she adds oils and perfumes purchased at a *botánica* to enhance the power of the *baño*. The final step is to light a candle over the *baño*. The candle is carefully balanced on a knife chosen for its convenience (to hold the candle) as well as for its mimetic powers (fig. 2.4).[7] As she lays the knife across the dish, she says, "This will help Ariel cut through obstacles he's got in his life." After lighting the candle, Jerusalén silently and quickly recites a blessing and snaps her fingers over the flame three times. When the candle burns out, the energized *baño* is filtered into a repurposed plastic bottle and is given to her grandson with explicit instructions for use (fig. 2.5).

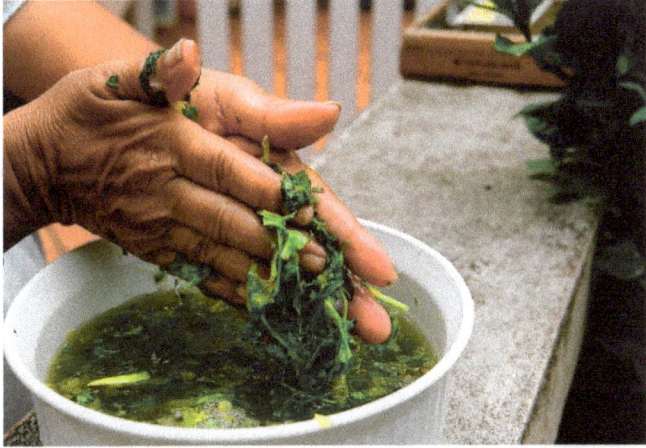

Fig. 2.3. Jerusalén uses her hands to crush a bird of paradise bud into rainwater. *Photograph by Selina Morales, 2006.*

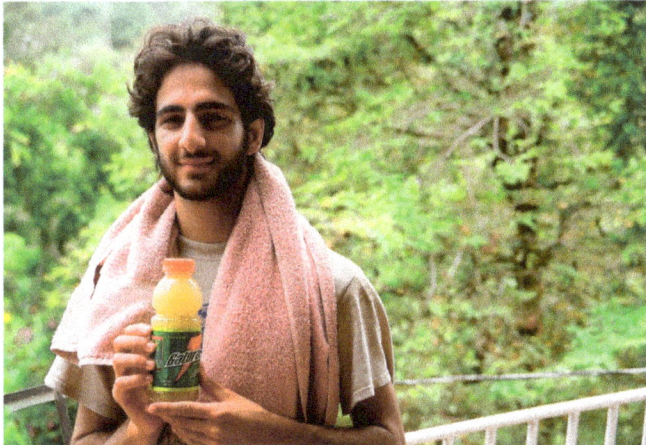

Fig. 2.4. Jerusalén lights a candle to enhance the power of her homemade baño. *Photograph by Selina Morales, 2006.*

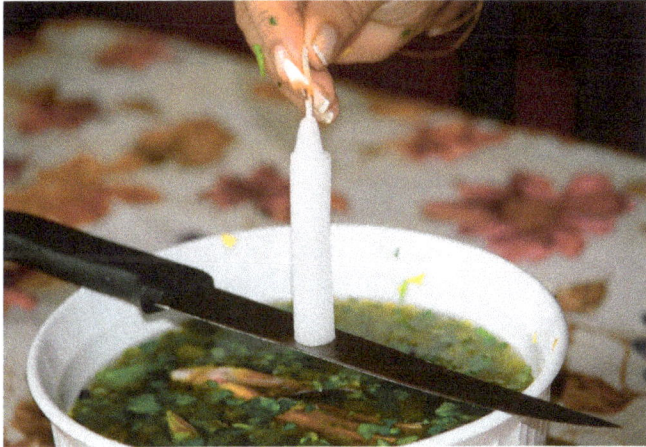

Fig. 2.5. Ariel Morales holds a bottle filled with a healing baño in Naranjito, Puerto Rico. *Photograph by Selina Morales, 2006.*

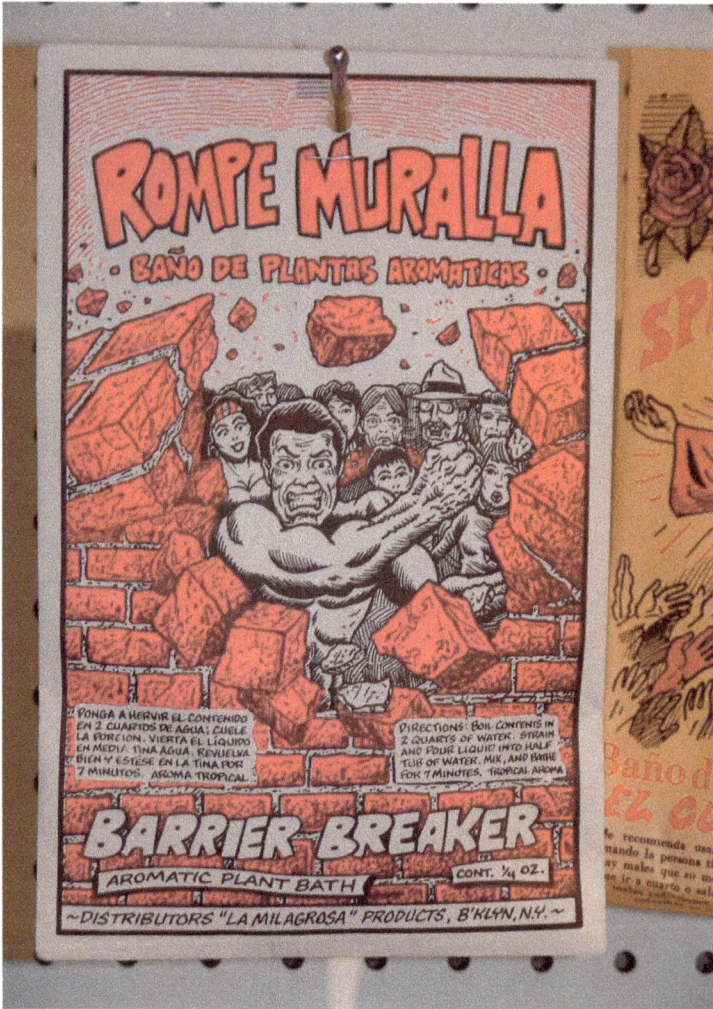

Fig. 2.6. Rompe Muralla/Barrier Breaker Aromatic Plant Bath, accession number 2010-08-0049, Mathers Museum of World Cultures, Indiana University. *Photograph by Selina Morales, 2008.*

In 1993, Jerusalén moved with her husband, Pedro Jaime Morales, from New York City to a rural farm nestled in the mountains south of San Juan, Puerto Rico. She rose to the challenge of continuing her business as a psychic and healer by quickly adapting her practices. On her tropical farm, she was able to harness natural elements to create spiritual remedies, supplementing as needed from *botánicas* on the island. After more than twenty years as a professional urban healer, the tools of her trade shifted in nuanced ways.

For example, consider this prepackaged *baño* (fig. 2.6). It is similar to those sold in *botánicas* in New York since the 1980s. It can be used to help individuals break through barriers in their lives. Jerusalén sold hundreds of these prepackaged remedies, often careful to give her own particular instructions, and fully aware that her clients were choosing to purchase these manufactured remedies from her blessed hands because they believed this would impact the efficacy of their rituals. Her customers' faith in her grace followed her spirit work from urban to rural landscapes, confirming for her now-global community that her connection to the spirits was/is, indeed, quite powerful.

Jerusalén has been working as a spirit medium and psychic her entire adult life. Her critical community work maintains her well-being; it fosters her relationships with others, keeps her relevant and relied upon, and combats the loneliness that might arise as one ages in a mobile home community in central Florida. In 2014, she moved with her husband to St. Cloud, Florida. Jerusalén, again, adapted her business model: phone consultations increased, and she slowly expanded her clients to include friends and relatives of her lifelong customers. When her husband passed in 2014, after completing her mourning period, she increased her phone consultations, often taking calls through the night. Calls continue to come in, from New York (and the northeast region), Puerto Rico, and locally from St. Cloud, Kissimmee, and Orlando.

## Staying Useful

When I was a little girl, my grandmother had me count out one hundred pennies, and after she blessed them, I helped her wrap each one in a small piece of red cloth, tied with a white ribbon. At her *botánica*, we sold each "lucky penny" for a dollar. Thirty years later, in 2016, I help her sort through a pail of loose change at my home in Philadelphia. We pick out one hundred pennies and bless and wrap them as we update each other about our lives. I am lucky. Jerusalén is visiting clients in Philadelphia, Delaware, New Jersey, and New York, and she uses my home as a base for the month. Her return to the Northeast is celebrated by many, and there is never enough time. Clients-turned-friends/family throw her parties, introduce her to their friends, show her the fruits of her labor (homes purchased, babies born, jobs landed) and widen her own networks. In between these visits, we work to prepare remedies, arrange her next consultations, or she follows through on promised prayers.

On this same visit, one of her clients and their friends have commissioned a dozen "magic pillows." Jerusalén spends her evenings hand sewing white lace onto the edges of brightly colored miniature pillows. Then, well after my household is asleep for the night, she makes the pillows magical. She imbues them with her grace, through prayer, perfume, and using her own powerful hands. She explains:

> Some people cannot sleep well, not because they have insomnia; some people do not sleep well because they have so many things going on in their brain that don't let them be calm and bring the time for themselves to rest for the next day. When I make the magic pillow, I [envision] that when this person lays on this pillow, their brain will be calmed down so they can have a better dream and they can see their future. Instead of being worried about the future, they can review and resolve problems that they have on their mind. It is not so much the perfume that I put [that makes the pillow work], but the energy that I drop with my hands on those pillows. The words that you speak are stronger than perfume . . . your words so strong that the pillow can [even] make you happy. And at the time to go to bed, you rest peacefully, and you have pleasant dreams about exactly what you want to have in life. (Jerusalén Morales, age eighty-five)

After all of these years, she is still concerned with others, concentrating on keeping them well. Retirement is not on her horizon. This past decade, with more than a hundred thousand Puerto Ricans migrating to Florida, there has been no lack of work for Jerusalén. And after Hurricane Maria devastated the island in 2017, it is expected that central Florida's Puerto Rican population will grow exponentially. And as she explains, working keeps her well, too:

> I am alone here, and I think, "What am I doing? I am not important anymore because I have no one." But when [my clients] call me, it is like a light to my brain. I can still be useful; I can help others. That is the way I see it; I feel very happy when they call me and they give me good and bad news. I am glad when they give me bad news; you know why? Because at the moment they are crying, I also see that they are changing; that pain they have in that moment is the end of their suffering. And when they finish talking, they say, "I don't know what to tell you, because I am a different person. I feel happy." It is amazing what goes on in my heart. I can help that person, and now she is happy, she is not angry anymore, she is not in pain anymore, and that makes me very happy.
>
> And after I hear all of that, I look at my life and I say, "My life is beautiful because there are other people who need me. . . . I can tell them at least a word that can change their life. I feel that I am useful, and [I] give my knowledge to the people. I can keep teaching and learning. Sometimes one word can change your life forever. (Jerusalén Morales, age eighty-six)

Selina Morales is Director of the Philadelphia Folklore Project and teaches in the Masters of Cultural Sustainability program at Goucher College.

## Works Cited

Harwood, Alan. 1987. *Rx Spiritist as Needed: A Study of a Puerto Rican Community Mental Health Resource*. Ithaca, NY: Cornell University Press.

Hurston, Zora Neale. 1935. *Mules and Men*. New York: Harper Perennial.

Kirshenblatt, Mayer, and Barbara Kirshenblatt-Gimblett. 2007. *They Called Me Mayer July*. Berkeley: University of California Press.

McCarthy Brown, Karen. 2001. *Mama Lola: A Vodou Priestess in Brooklyn*. Los Angeles: University of California Press.

Murphy, Joseph M. 1993. *Santería: African Spirits in America*. Boston: Beacon.

———. 2010. "Objects that Speak Creole: Juxtapositions of Shrine Devotions at Botanicas in Washington, DC." *Material Religion: The Journal of Objects, Art and Belief* 6 (March): 86–108.

———. 2015. *Botánicas: Sacred Spaces of Healing and Devotion in Urban America*. Jackson: University Press of Mississippi.

Myerhoff, Barbara. 1978. *Number Our Days: A Triumph of Continuity and Culture among Jewish Old People in an Urban Ghetto*. New York: Simon & Schuster.

Polk, Patrick, ed. 2004. *Botánica Los Angeles: Latino Popular Religious Art in the City of Angels*. Los Angeles: Fowler Museum of Cultural History, University of California, Los Angeles.

Romberg, Raquel. 2003. *Witchcraft and Welfare Spiritual Capital and the Business of Magic in Modern Puerto Rico*. Austin: University of Texas Press.

Trinh T. Minh-ha. 1989. *Woman, Native, Other*. Bloomington: Indiana University Press.

## Notes

1. *Espiritismo*, as a belief system with doctrine and rules, has been defined in books. However, in my lifetime of participating in communities of "practitioners" and my eighteen years of formally interviewing individuals about their practices, I have yet to meet a person who relies on a formal definition or doctrine when describing what this belief system entails. Here is what Jerusalén explains: *Espiritistas*, or people who practice *espiritismo*, share the belief that metaphysical spirits influence people's lives. The human body is a vehicle or vessel for these spirits or souls. When a person dies, their spirit is released back into the spirit realm and, likely, reborn. Jerusalén says, "We are souls more than anything," and uses Catholicism's guardian angels in order to exemplify the place spirits have in the world. For further reading on *espiritismo* and *brujería*, see Harwood 1987 and Romberg 2003, respectively.

2. Grace is Jerusalén's English word for her ability to heal others; in Spanish, she says *bendición*. The communication of grace is metaphysical; we cannot see grace, but it is her grace that heals others.

3. Jerusalén tells and retells this story often. This 2001 version features Oshun, an Orisha/spirit/deity worshiped throughout the African diaspora by practitioners of diverse African-rooted belief systems (see Murphy 1993 for an accessible review of Santería's history and pantheon of deities). Details in this origin story vary from telling to telling; the last time I heard this story was in 2017. At eighty-six years old, Jerusalén recounted this to her two daughters and all of her granddaughters as we enjoyed lunch in her home. At that time, she further elaborated on the problems that caused her blindness, rather than on what she did as a result of gaining a third eye (as she does in the next part of the 2001

interview). What stories do women tell one another at different stages of life? A question for the tellers and for the listeners.

4. According to Jerusalén, at the stroke of midnight on La Noche de San Juan, the waters surrounding Puerto Rico become blessed and possess special powers. Puerto Ricans from all over the island flock to San Juan, the island's capital, to bath in the ocean at midnight. Traditionally, there are bonfires on the beach and live music. At midnight, people walk backward into the water to receive the blessing from San Juan. The blessing is said to cure sickness, give beauty, improve fortune, aid in fertility, increase agricultural production, and ward off evil. My grandmother claims that if you submerge yourself in water at midnight, you will receive prophesizing dreams of your year to come: a chance for ordinary people to experience psychic powers for a limited time.

5. Jerusalén owned a *botánica*, or store that sells ritual objects, in the South Bronx, where she both sold these objects and gave consultations. For further reading about *botánicas*, see Murphy 2010, 2015; Polk 2004; and Romberg 2003).

6. Jerusalén clarifies: "Prayer is not only the Our Father; prayer should be something that is in your mind that you are giving away of yourself for another person, and a good thought will penetrate because it is something very powerful, the thoughts that you have. That is why I cannot see your thoughts and you cannot see mine, because they are so powerful."

7. Ritual objects often have mimetic powers as they may stand for metaphysical ideas. A rose, or even the color red, could stand for love. The flower called *mira-mi-linda*, or "look at me, I'm pretty," can make you stand out or even beautiful. Jerusalén recognizes the power of mimesis and incorporates it into her healing work.

# 3     Fieldworker in the Cane

## A Puerto Rican Life History in Wood and Words

### Julián Antonio Carrillo

A T NINETY-THREE, JOSÉ Lugo Arroyo is many things: a woodcarver, painter, poet, chronicler, and novelist, as well as a retired soldier, teacher, mathematician, and university administrator. Most importantly, perhaps, he is also a *jíbaro* in mind and soul—a small farmer in Puerto Rico, typically from a mountainous region.[1] Having recently *convivido* with him in his rural Virginia home, I am adding "ethnographic fieldworker" to his list of occupations.[2]

In 1974, Sidney Mintz published *Worker in the Cane: A Puerto Rican Life History*, which presents the life of don "Taso" Zayas, a sugarcane worker who, like his peers in the 1930s and 1940s, was impacted by the socioeconomic changes brought on by westernization.[3] Don Taso's life history serves, as Mintz (1974, ix–xii) puts it, as a testament to a superbly intelligent man as well as to his drastically changing society. This chapter presents the life of don José Lugo Arroyo, who like don Taso, labored in the Puerto Rican countryside during a similar time of transformation. Yet, here I focus on his artwork.

Before leaving the island at the age of eighteen to serve in World War II in 1943, don José lived the first part of his life in rural Puerto Rico where he experienced, learned about, and documented vernacular practices all around him. Much later as an adult, don José began to recollect those experiences and materialize his memories in a collection of handcrafted wooden figurines documenting the rich diversity of Puerto Rican folklife of the 1930s and 1940s.[4]

Based on the nature and content of his woodcarvings, I label don José a folkloristic ethnographic fieldworker and his carved scenes an "ethnographic" collec-

*The Expressive Lives of Elders* (2018): 55–79, DOI: 10.2979/expressivelivesofelders.0.0.04

tion.[5] Parting from this premise, this chapter asks the following questions: Why does the need to carve ethnographic sculptures become a necessity later in the life of don José? What is involved in his woodcarving, and why does the creative process become an activity in its own right? Moreover, how do the sculptures acquire value?

To answer these questions, the chapter looks at how don José's condition as a fieldworker involved a creative process that was based on the mobilization of memory in various ways. This chapter also explores the ways that the intimate value of his collection has grown throughout the years to acquire greater value as heritage. Last, I show that as folklorists we have something to offer elders if we highlight and work from the intra- and intergenerational connections, which are crucial to the valorization of their folk arts.

## Expressions in Wood

Don José currently resides with his daughter Sonia Ivette Badillo and her husband, Leslie Elvis Badillo, in a house nestled in the thick woods surrounding the town of Christiansburg, Virginia. The many rooms of this country home are dotted with evidence of how proud this strong family is of its Puerto Rican heritage. The halls are adorned with photographs of the Badillos' three adult sons, Walter, Brian, and Alex, next to paintings of their parents' and grandparents' cherished Island of Enchantment.

The first thing we see when we enter the room dedicated to don José's collection, which he calls Expressions in Wood, is a white wall with symmetrically placed shelves. These hold one hundred hand-painted sculptures, some of which are a few inches tall while others are so large that they must be picked up with both hands. Collectively, the carvings make up an entire colorful village of miniature people, all engaged in activity (fig. 3.1).

Some of these villagers are at home tending a fire on a traditional stove with sand, wood, and rocks; feeding their children or husbands; or sitting on a small wooden bench patiently rolling tobacco. Other people's work extends outward to the barrio, like the barber cutting a man's hair under a palm tree or the man selling *piraguas* (snow cones) from his little cart. A few kids play games. One, for example, is on the street with *la rueda*, rolling a metallic wheel without letting it fall over. Country folk are also portrayed in the midst of the daily grind—fishing, hauling jugs of water, carrying lumber, cutting open coconuts with their machetes, and working the *caña* (sugarcane), either alone or with the help of oxen. In contrast, there are those who prefer to play dice or place their bets down for a cockfight. In one corner of the room sits a *bohío* (a traditional house) on stilts, with an outhouse and a triangular, low-lying *tormentera* (storm shelter) in the back; its homeowner stands by the door, watching her chickens in the front yard while her little pig eats near a tree stump (fig. 3.2).

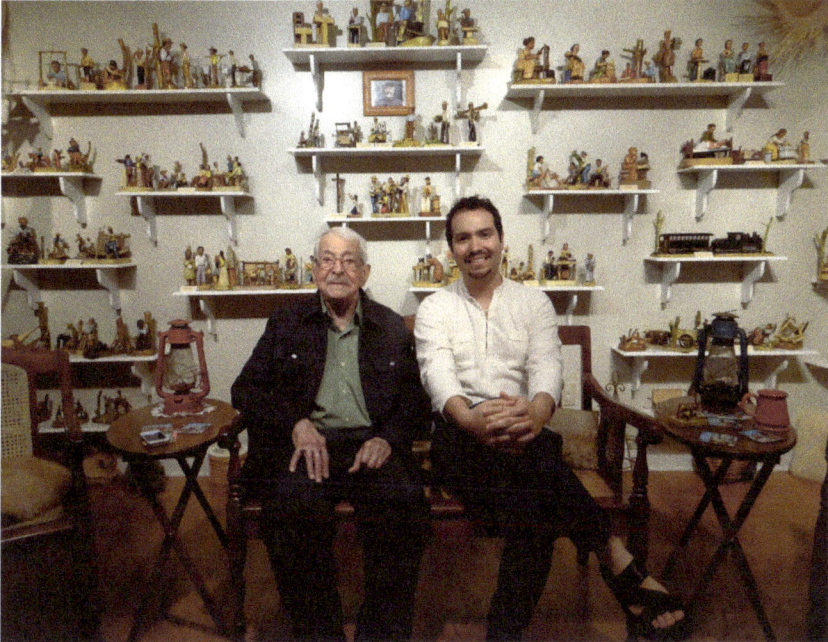

Fig. 3.1. Don José and the author in front of the collection, 2017.
*Courtesy of Sonia Ivette Badillo.*

Track lighting installed overhead gives the room and the pieces a curatorial ambience, while tiny labels on the shelves organize the collection by themes: "Crabbing," "Traditional pig roast," "Coconut drink," "Shaved ice treat," "Saw and piglets," "Jíbaro house," "Clandestine still," "Milking the cow," "Steam locomotive," "Working the land," "Motherhood," "Women at work," "Puerto Rican pastime," "Doing chores," "Working the sugarcane," "Connecting with God," "Good old days," "Working a trade," "Family life," "Social life," "Men at work," "The Jíbaro," "Gone fishing," and "Rest and relaxation."

I met don José when I visited the Badillos in June 2017.[6] Leslie—tall, dark haired, and handsome with an easy smile—is a Puerto Rican–born doctor who has been practicing in Christiansburg for more than twenty-five years. Sonia—tall, svelte, soft spoken, and kind—is also originally from Puerto Rico. She is a housewife and an aerobics instructor at the Christiansburg Recreation Center, where she works with seniors.

After we introduced ourselves, I looked to my left and saw don José standing there—strong and upright—with the aid of his newly acquired walker. I approached him, extended my hand, and noticing his calm and thoughtful gaze, said, smiling, "It's a pleasure to meet you," in Spanish. Hearing me perfectly well,

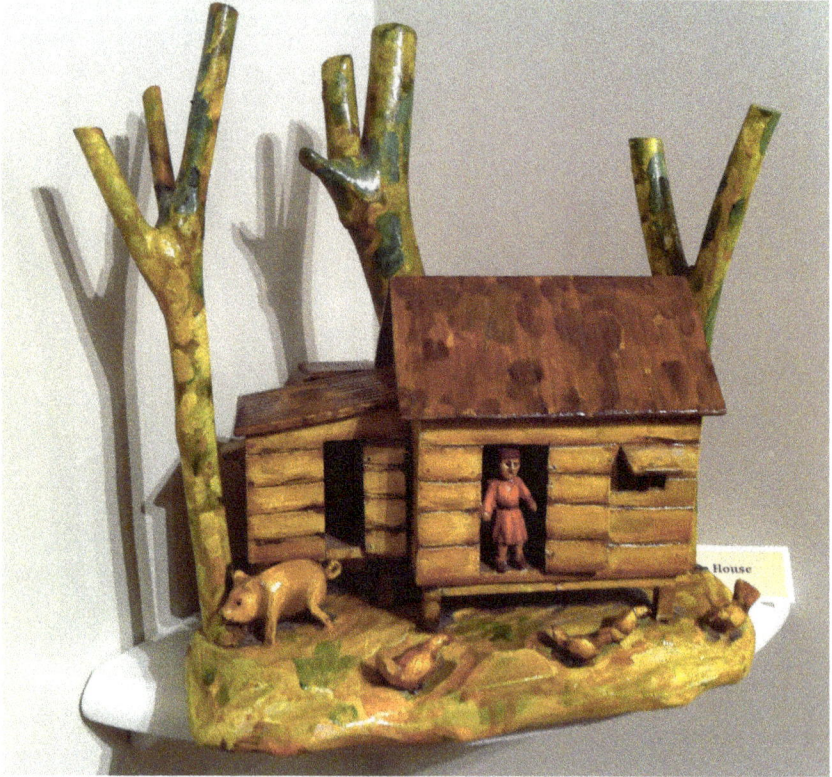

Fig. 3.2. A traditional Puerto Rican rural house, 2017. *Photograph by Julián Antonio Carrillo.*

he responded, *"Igualmente."*[7] That evening—after a dinner consisting of white rice, *habichuelas* (beans), and fried plantains—don José agreed to show me his collection.

"These are the figures. I have carved ninety-eight of them," he said as we entered the room. He then showed me a boy milking a cow while a calf looks on. "This is the first one" (fig. 3.3). Sonia brought a second example, the same figure of a male milking a cow and a calf observing him (fig. 3.4), only this time the "boy" had a receding hairline and the piece was more detailed and colorful. This was a remake, they told me, of the first piece but many years later with more expertise. I would later come to learn that both of these figurines represent don José, one of his many childhood memories.

Considering the above, I posit that "Expressions" constitutes a collection of ethnographic "memory objects." A memory object is an item created "as a way to materialize internal images, and through them, to recapture earlier experiences.

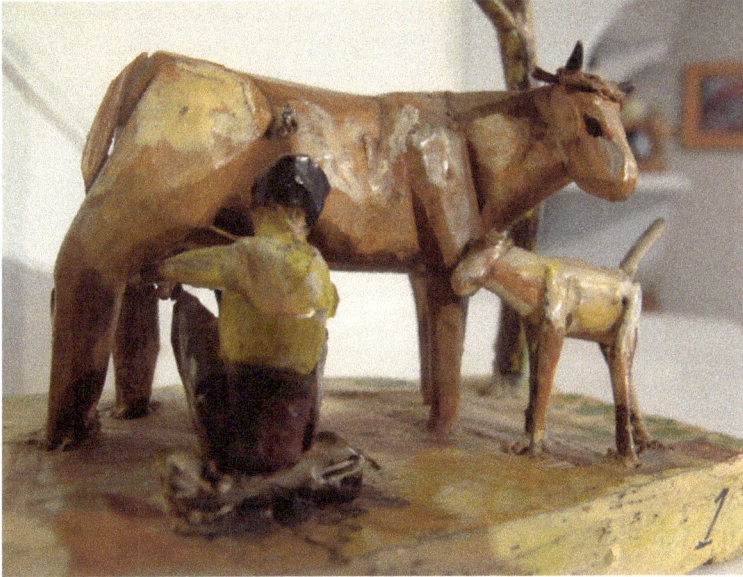

Fig. 3.3. Don José's first memory object in his collection, 2017. *Photograph by Julián Antonio Carrillo.*

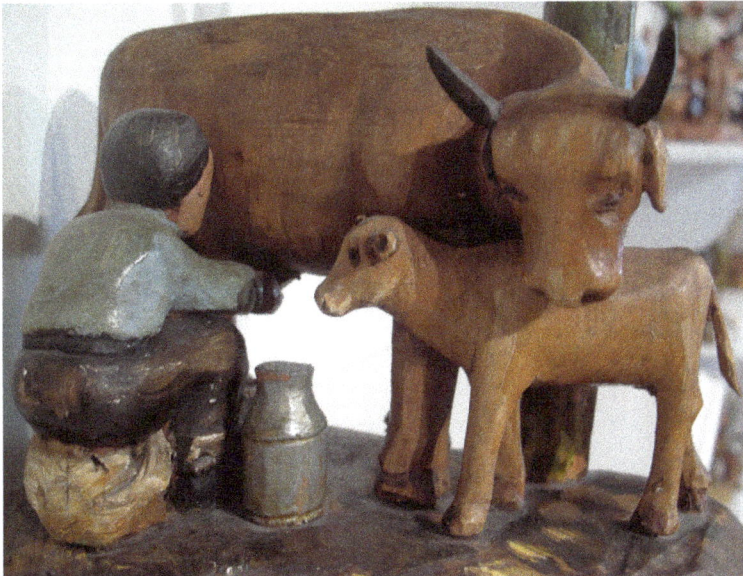

Fig. 3.4. A remake, years later, of don José's first memory object in his collection, 2017. *Photograph by Julián Antonio Carrillo.*

Whereas souvenirs are saved prospectively, with a sense of their future ability to call back memories, memory objects are produced retrospectively, long after the events they depict transpired" (Kirshenblatt-Gimblett 1985, 331). These creations also have the capacity to serve "as tools for reviewing and sharing personal stories, and provide a catalyst for conversations and social interactions" (Kay 2016, 6; Kirshenblatt-Gimblett 1985, 336). For don José, then, each wooden figurine that he created is a memory (or several) that he imbues with significance. However, some have more meaning than others; don José refers to these as "intimate":

> All of them are significant and mean something to me. But there are some that I like because they are intimate. For example, that figure in which a woman is blowing into a kettle. It is hard for me to let go of that figure because it reminds me of my mother. . . . And there is another one that I also remember a great deal which is the one depicting the dance, that one was a memory of my aunt [Rafaela, a devotee of the three saints], who would go out with the *parranda* [days] before [Epiphany] to celebrate. . . . She would [host a yearly gathering at her house in addition to visiting all the neighborhood] houses, [with] musicians. . . . [It] reminds me of a great deal. . . . It has much value for me.[8]

At eight years old, don José began to experience his aunt Rafaela's festivities, which accounts for the *parranda*'s intimate meaning (fig. 3.5). He recalls, for instance, writing lyrics to *música de aguinaldo*, which he would give to his aunt who, in turn, would pass along to the local musicians performing from house to house.[9]

But these carvings not only hold personal, intimate value. Even don José acknowledges that they reflect everyday social life on the island in a specific historic moment: "[My artwork is] a project of woodcarvings of scenes from my barrio and hometown, which naturally, were also common scenes of the daily life of other barrios and towns in Puerto Rico and probably similar to other places in other countries as well. . . . These were scenes of things I lived and that were part of my daily life. They were saved in my memory. In a way, they are a reflection of the socioeconomic conditions in which we, the country men [*campesinos* or peasants], lived between the years of 1900–1945." Indeed, his carvings reflect what don José witnessed in and around his hometown of Quebradillas. The cultural practices depicted in wood have either changed or are no longer performed in large part because of the historical changes brought on by capitalism in the mid-twentieth century.[10] As the above quote suggests, don José was a "participant observer" in/to these changes.

While the figurines speak for themselves in many ways, don José speaks through them or with them, as my first personal encounter with his art reveals. That evening in front of the collection, he led me to the left corner of the wall, pointed toward a shelf whose label read "Gone Fishing" and said, "We will begin here. The figures at the top are the *jueyeros* or crab hunters . . . [they work] with

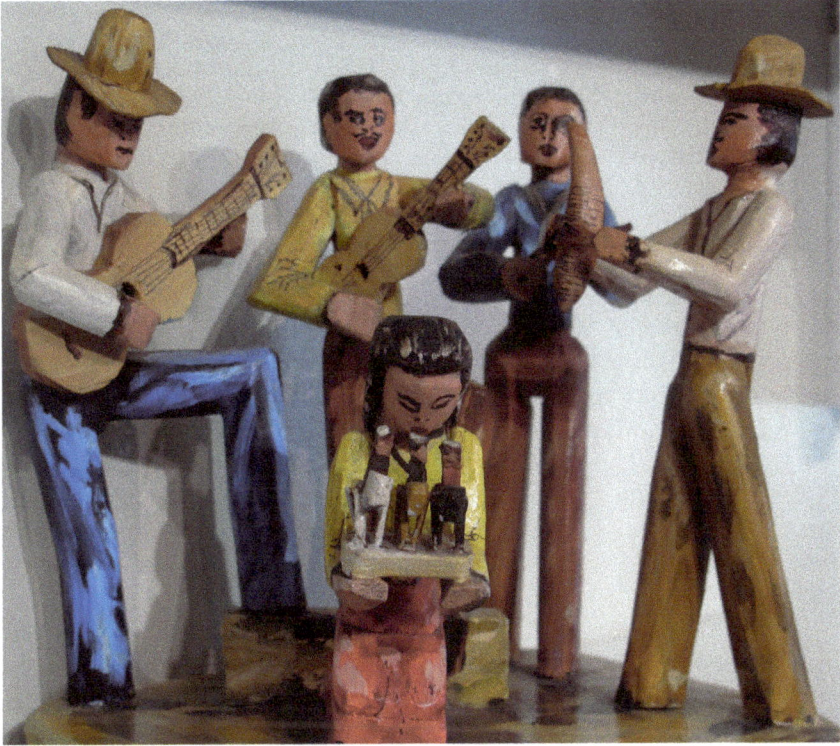

Fig. 3.5. "La Parranda," 2017. *Photograph by Julián Antonio Carrillo.*

their hands . . . they know how to catch them." That is, he shared with me the traditional knowledge that these villagers once had. He also taught me about historical change, in this case the effects of the collapse of the sugarcane industry in the mid-1960s: "Let me tell you that down there in Puerto Rico there are no more crabs. Now they have to import them from Santo Domingo [the Dominican Republic] because the crab, the *juey* as we call them, lived amongst the cane, the sugarcane. Since there is no more cane, the *jueyes* have also ceased to exist. . . . They say [sugarcane] was not economically productive enough to [survive]." In this sense, each of these ethnographic scenes serve, as memory objects often do, to share "personal stories, and provide a catalyst for conversations and social interactions" (Kay 2016, 6; Kirshenblatt-Gimblett 1985, 336), only in this case, they elicit ethnographic data about a particular social group.[11]

Nevertheless, what gave birth to such a large and long-term woodcarving project? Was it just don José's desire to recall and document his lived experience? On one hand, don José answers these questions very simply and directly:

Since my childhood, I have always felt a special admiration for art and I have been attracted to sculpture, painting, and carving . . . [even though I had to work when I was young,] I [still] entertained myself and fulfilled my creative desires by carving figures of workers and the tools they used to accomplish their tasks. Then I would give them away or throw them away. . . . [Even as an adult I continued to toss what I would carve] . . . this whole thing concerning the figures [that I began to collect] came to me for no specific reason. I would carve them and then I would discard them somewhere. . . . Delia, this is the work of [my wife] Delia. She said [to me], "Give me these things instead; I'm going to keep them."

With this request from his late wife, doña Delia Esther Lorenzo Veintidós, indeed don José began to keep everything he carved from that moment onward, as they became gifts for his loving wife. While she played a key role in starting and safeguarding this collection, which we will explore later, on closer inspection the value that she bestowed on the woodcarvings does not explain the entire story. As we shall see, a more complete answer lies in the creative process that brought these figurines into existence. However, in order to understand this process, we first need to contextualize it in relation to don José's life history, to which I turn next.[12]

Two periods are key in the following life history narrative: don José's "formative period" when he was a boy living in rural Puerto Rico and his "retirement period" when, as a married adult, he returned to live in a rural setting after having spent time abroad and working in urban areas. As I aim to show later, these two periods "converged" in don José's creative process informing or feeding off of each other as he readapted to living in rural Puerto Rico; thus, "Expressions" is a product of this convergence.

## A Concise History of a Long Life

Don José was born on January 15, 1925, in the town of Quebradillas, whose inhabitants dedicated themselves to small-scale agricultural production—particularly beans, corn, tobacco, and cotton. Specifically, he grew up in a section of the barrio Terranova that was known as Quebrada Mala. Of this setting that enveloped his formative period, he avidly remembers "the entanglement of neighborhood pathways that the local youth and I would roam; the games at night that we would invent to take advantage of the clarity of a full moon; the gatherings under the palm groves from which we could scan in the distance the horizontal line where the ocean and sky are confused in a leaden embrace. That was my microcosm."

Don José was part of a numerous family with humble beginnings. The oldest of eight siblings, he lived in crowded, temporary makeshift houses, and his parents, Dolores "Mamá Lola" Arroyo and José Lugo, worked hard to make ends

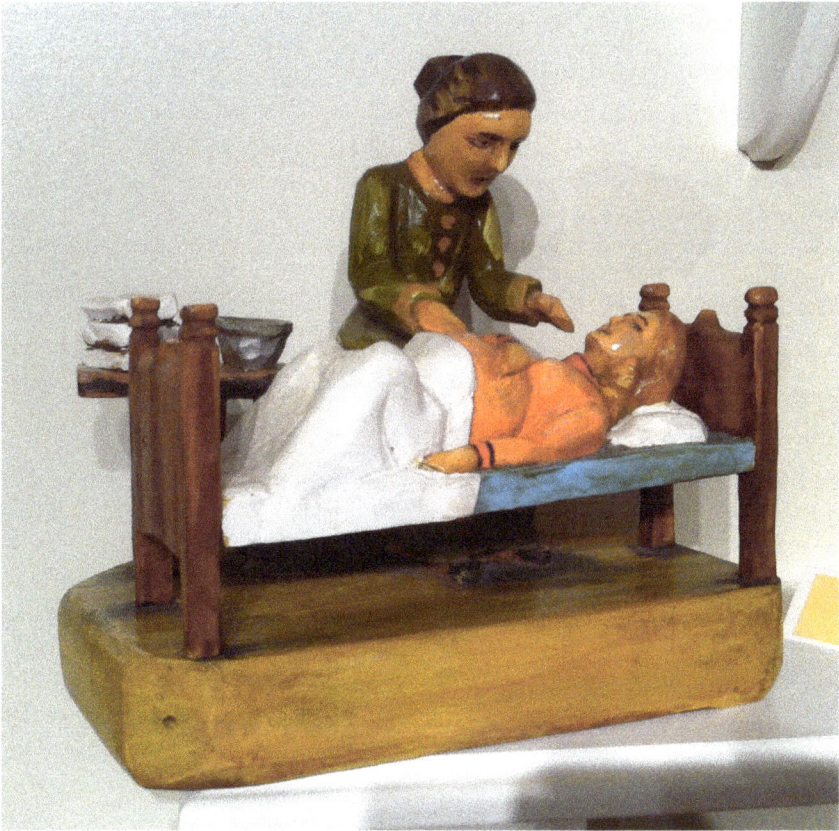

Fig. 3.6. "La Partera," a carving depicting don José's paternal grandmother, 2017. *Photograph by Julián Antonio Carrillo.*

meet. His father earned a living as an agricultural laborer. His mother took care of the household. Despite the shortages and socioeconomic hardships, don José states that "we felt happy and we were raised free."

Don José was particularly close to his paternal grandparents. His grandmother, Juana Gandía, was a highly solicited *partera* (midwife) and healer (fig. 3.6). He remembers accompanying her as early as age six: "I would wait outside the room where she was working and sometimes fall asleep in a corner. When you would hear the baby crying . . . that is when you knew Grandma was coming out and it was time to go home." He also remembers her large garden from which she would pick flowers and plants to make herbal remedies; "she could fix a headache with sage and a *santiguo*."[13] Her front porch, he reminisces, was the neighborhood social hub—people would gather on Sundays to talk, eat, drink, and dance to music from an old Victrola.[14]

As for don José's paternal grandfather, Telésforo Lugo, he was a common hardworking peasant who knew a great deal about the art of tobacco making. As a kid, don José frequently accompanied him to the fields. Other times, when Grandpa went to town to the casino, he would give his grandson money to go see western and Mexican films at the cinema.

As a young man, don José focused on his studies and on entering the workforce, even though he would have preferred to study art. This sacrifice was paramount because in the midst of the Great Depression, scarcity and economic limitations intensified with each passing day. As he states, "It seemed there was no end to the condition of misery in which we lived. . . . In the period of my development as a [young] person, there were socioeconomic situations that directed me toward other priorities and urgencies that demanded the attention in that moment. . . . In those days, I had no means to study that which I liked [art], so I dedicated my time first to working, then to studying, with the goal of preparing myself to immediately enter the labor market."

In 1939, he graduated from eighth grade, and even though he wanted to continue studying, he needed to contribute to his household. During this period, he labored in *fincas* (farms), built houses, and chiseled stones for the construction of modern roads earning a dollar a day. His "big break" arrived when he became a "tow truck operator" at the nearby train station—where his dad and uncle worked temporarily—packaging and shipping sugarcane for forty dollars a month.

In 1942, he was drafted into the US Army and left the island for the first time. He was stationed in a military base near Colón, Panama, where, as part of the 761st AAA Gun Battalion, he trained soldiers in artillery. In between intense periods of work, he would play the guitar and sing for his army compatriots.

In 1946, after being discharged, don José returned to Puerto Rico where he enrolled in ninth grade in Quebradillas. In 1949, he graduated high school in Isabela and, thanks to the GI Bill, was able to enroll in the Programa Normal del Colegio de Pedagogía of the University of Puerto Rico (UPR), Rio Piedras campus.

On the first day of college, don José met his future wife, doña Delia, who was also starting in the same teaching program. They became good friends, spending a great deal of time together. Eventually, toward the end of college, he proposed and doña Delia gladly accepted.

In 1952, after graduation and marriage, the newlyweds worked as teachers in Quebradillas. This began what would ultimately become a lifelong career path for both individuals, serving in various teaching and administrative positions—sometimes at the same schools or universities—until don José and doña Delia retired in 1980 and 1985, respectively.

Between the beginning and end of their careers, don José and doña Delia raised three daughters—Sylvia Enid (b. 1953), Sonia Ivette (b. 1959), and Carmen Delia (b. 1962). While family life was always central to the couple, they welcomed every opportunity to develop professionally, adapting to challenging circumstances when required.

For instance, from 1960 to 1961 don José participated and completed an academic course in mathematics for secondary school teachers at UPR, under the auspices of the National Science Foundation. Similarly, in 1964, doña Delia began a master's program in special education at the University of Illinois, Urbana-Champaign. This required the family to move to and adapt to the Midwest.

While certainly a trying time, don José describes living in Urbana as unforgettable. There, don José took care of the girls, prepared meals, and maintained the household while his wife finished her master's and started her doctorate. He took this opportunity to teach himself how to paint through the aid of course materials, which he received on a monthly basis by mail. He later painted many portraits in addition to some Puerto Rican landscapes. (Later as a retiree, he would employ these skills in "Expressions.")

In Urbana, the couple—strongly rooted in the Presbyterian Church—formed a supportive community, made friends, and created lifelong bonds. Abroad, don José also worked as engineering assistant in the Department of Hydraulic Engineering of the US Department of Agriculture's Soil Conservation Services. In 1966, doña Delia concluded her master's and doctoral studies, and the couple returned to Puerto Rico.

In 1967, now living in the San Juan metropolitan area, doña Delia began to teach as a professor in the newly created Special Education Program in the College of Pedagogy at UPR, a position she held for twenty years until she retired. During her tenure, she also served three years as the director of the Escuela Superior of UPR.

As for don José, in his last few years before retirement, he held a variety of positions—including math teacher in the Escuela Superior Sotero Figueroa, auxiliary scientific researcher at the Center for Pedagogical Research at UPR, statistics coordinator in the Office of Planning and Research at UPR, and director of the Division of Statistics of the Central Administration of the Office of the President of UPR.

As early as 1974, don José had several "post-retirement" projects and objectives in mind that, while dormant, roamed his mind for years looking for the opportunity to manifest. Among these, he states, "I wanted to carve Puerto Rican figures in wood; paint landscapes, which is something I always enjoyed; read books that slept in a corner waiting for their moment; and above all, I yearned to have a place where I could grow crops, farm, and be close to nature."

In 1985, thanks to doña Delia's acceptance, these wishes came true when the couple moved to Loma Vista, a *finca* in rural Trujillo Alto, Puerto Rico. It was during this "retirement period" that don José created the bulk of "Expressions."

In 2007, the couple moved from the *finca* to Quebradillas to a house that doña Delia could manage better. Then in 2010, they had to migrate to the United States to live with the Badillos because don José suffered a hemorrhagic stroke and could not properly care for his wife, who was suffering from Alzheimer's. Also, he underwent open-heart surgery in the United States for an aortic valve replacement but thankfully recovered well. In 2016, doña Delia unfortunately passed away. Don José continues to live in Christiansburg in the care of his family.

## The Creative Process: Mobilizations of Memory

How does carving fit into the above life history narrative? Why did don José want to "carve Puerto Rican figures in wood" as a "postretirement" project? The answer lies in the creative process that brought his collection into existence.

Jon Kay states that elders reach a point in their lives where creativity bursts and they create looking toward the past in an engagement with a "life review" process, which makes art so powerful at this age. This art can be so potent that it serves to inspire future conversations and other narratives once it has been created and the social life of the art has begun. Kay writes, "the combined processes of seniors reviewing their lives, making art based on this reflection, and narrating their creations for others is a distinctive and widespread phenomenon that deserves more attention." In particular, we need to "appreciate the complex and diverse narrative nature of these creations and *the process that brought them into existence*" (Kay 2016, 5–6, emphasis added).

I argue that the period in don José's life leading up to retirement, retirement itself, and the subsequent accompanying move that he and his wife made from an urban setting to a rural one marks his initial "life review" period and that "Expressions" is the result of submerging himself in his life review.[15] In this process, several operations that I call mobilizations of memory converge: Identification, Compare and Contrast, and Memory Transfer. In each of these, memory is operationalized, deployed, or sparked *in different ways*, serving a different function.

### Identification

In the 1960s in Illinois, don José learned to paint and did so regularly, but he never painted any of the ethnographic scenes that he would later carve in the 1980s. He didn't do so because "in Urbana there was another environment. I adapted to the environment that was there. . . . [Painting] was one more adaptation that I did [in my life]. . . . Because it was something else, it was Urbana, a town. And we have to adapt to the town where we live." This quote seems to suggest that don José feels that "you should bloom where you are planted"—that is, adapt to the new "soil" in which you live and thrive.

Moreover, even when don José admits, laughing, that sometimes in Urbana he felt a desire to "grab a knife" and carve, he didn't do it because "it was not the [right] moment" ("*no era el momento*"). In fact, he never wanted to paint the *jíbaro* because the *jíbaro* was his "own" ("*el jíbaro era cosa mía*"), something that he carries inside him. As he replied when I asked him about these matters: "Why am I going to paint him when I can carve him? For each [artistic] medium there is an adaptation . . . that must be made. . . . That other stuff [painting] was not mine. . . . [Maybe if I had learned to paint since I was a child] painting [as an artistic medium] would be mine . . . [but I was only its] student. The same thing happened with writing; I had to make an adaptation when I went to college. . . . [I had to learn to write, and through practice] now it is mine." Don José's responses to my questions are insightful. His response, "it was not the [right] moment" indexes that it was not yet his time to begin his life review, but it also reveals how carving, as opposed to painting or even writing, is constitutive of his identity as a "*jíbaro*."

In other words, the specificity of the artistic medium (carving) matters because he associates it with his sense of self, he remembers it is a part of who he is. In this regard, the medium, the form, and the content—all three elements—constitute part of don José's identity as a *jíbaro*. This is not surprising as the following written autobiographical quote shows that he learned a great deal from his folk:

> I am aware that among these facts no heroic deeds are told nor any figures of grand prominence with grand titles included, but there is an entire tradition, a culture, and some social features that defined a group of peasants. Authentic *jíbaros*, amongst which I was born and I *conviví* with for some time. Many of them were my models. From them I learned some values that have been my guide throughout the trajectory of my life. In particular: love for work, respect for people, honesty, fidelity to what is promised, sharing what one has with those who have the greatest needs, respect for nature, and attachment to family.

It is not surprising, then, that don José did not paint the *jíbaro* in Urbana as carving the *jíbaro*, not painting him, is something that he has always done since he was a *jíbaro* youth. It also makes sense that on returning physically and mentally (through his memories) to the rural space where he grew up, he would naturally take up an artistic practice that he had "left behind" while simultaneously, like the *jíbaro*, always carried inside him.

I argue that familiarity and identification with the medium of expression (the tools for carving), form (the woodcarvings, the result), and content (what these woodcarvings signify) is an operation that activated/used/sparked don José's memory. So once don José "rekindled" his relationship to carving—which he had not practiced regularly until he retired—it awoke even more memories because not only was he familiar with a medium, a form, or a content, but more importantly, perhaps, he identified with all three.

But what did carving in late age help him accomplish? As we shall see next, in the operation that I call Compare and Contrast, memory was deployed to make sense of his new rural environment and ultimately help him adapt to it.

## Compare and Contrast

Just like don José tells us that he adapted to Urbana, including taking up painting, I argue that he also adapted to the Puerto Rico that he encountered in the 1980s after retirement, in part, through carving. I have already shown above how carving was constitutive to his identity as a *jíbaro*; here, I make the case that the process of carving during his life review period involved a second mobilization of memory: comparing and contrasting the environment he remembered from childhood with the environment he had retired to.

This subprocess of carving helped him, I argue, make sense of his "new" environment and ultimately adapt to it. That is, through the production of figurines, don José was actively trying to make sense of the changes around him in rural Puerto Rico of the 1980s and 1990s in order to adapt—essentially, asking himself, "Where do I 'fit in' in this environment that has changed so much since I last lived in it?" In part, then, he was "carving a niche" for himself.

As a boy, don José first absorbed, like an ethnographic fieldworker, the "folklore of his *pueblo*."[16] As he once told me, "Well, I carry it [the folklore of my pueblo] with me. How [this happened] I don't know; it stuck to me a long time ago, since I was a boy. I am a folklorist . . . and I like it." Also important in this process is that he carved these observations and experiences when they were still fresh in his young mind: "Of course. Yes. That [collection] is an entire memory what you have right there. I started it when I was a boy, I started in my neighborhood, as a boy, but as I have told you [before Julián], what I carved, well, it did not have much importance to me so I simply would toss it." Although he tossed his pieces, the practice of woodcarving had a significant effect: it served to ingrain in his mind these experiences to the point of remembering incredible detail.[17]

The memories of place, people, and cultural practices, of which some made into wooden form, have always accompanied don José throughout his life. However, on returning to live permanently in rural Puerto Rico after retirement, he began to compare and contrast that past way of life with the current (1980s and 1990s) environment. That is, from the point of view of his older self, don José was contrasting different places and times in the process of carving his collection.

In this context, don José was reliving in his mind what the countryside of his childhood that he had left thirty or forty years ago looked like, felt like, and smelled like, before "westernization" displaced those families and structures that had once structured his childhood and adolescence:

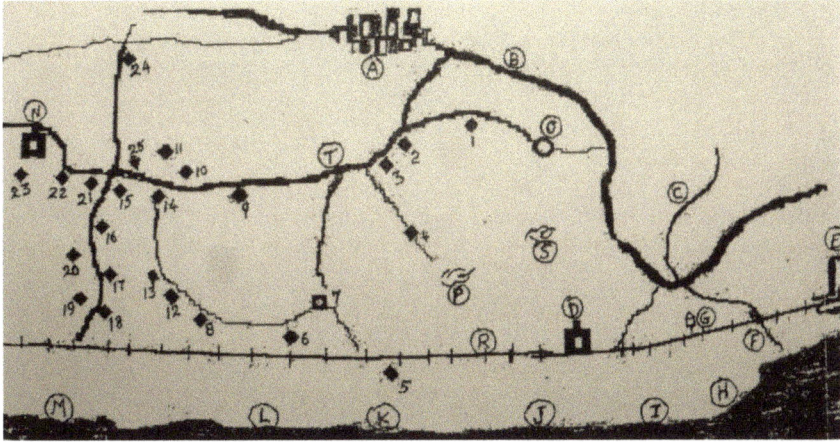

Fig. 3.7. Don José's mental map of his hometown, 2017. *Photograph courtesy of José Lugo Arroyo.*

This map does not respond to any parameters of any kind. It was drawn based on data that resides in my memory and its purpose is to situate the structures and the families where they were located between 1930 and 1945. In actuality, the panorama has completely changed. . . . Today, abrupt changes, the modality of consumerism, technological advances, and the eagerness for acquiring have all together ruined that little world. The families are no longer there; the old people have gone away. The little wooden or palm tree houses from yesteryear have vanished, substituted by mansions or big houses made of cement that seem to intimidate those that get too close. The labyrinth of worn-out little roads that appeared to travel from house to house, as if greeting people, no longer exists.

Moreover, I argue that *comparing* and *contrasting* these two "worlds"—the rural and the urban—don José was carving another dimension, another time and that this process was his trying to make sense of the socioeconomic changes while managing to adapt to them. This heightened sense of existential awareness—experienced by anyone who has ever left their hometown or region for a long time only to return to see it significantly changed—was fueling don José's carving. Perhaps that is why he is able to write and speak with such eloquence about what it feels like to see "progress" displace an entire social reality he once knew and documented:

Now everything is asphalt and gates that delimit every property as if saying, "Stop right there. From here on you shall not pass." Even the topography of the barrio has changed. The main alley that connected the barrio with the village and adjacent villages, turned into a road through which progress, taking advantage, came down displacing in its steps the reality of an epoch. . . . Oh, what hopes and dreams I remember from that stage [my microcosm, my child-hood neighborhood]! Things that time and succinct reality have taken care of erasing, or better said, of transforming into blurry shadows as my world broadened and other ideas were conceived.[18]

Interestingly, this "dismembered" Puerto Rican countryside caused by more visible manifestations of "private property" than before—with fences, gates, and signs that read, "Do not step on the grass," "No trespassing," or "Private prop-erty"—is "remembered" by don José in his collection and the stories he tells, fur-ther proof of his ethnographic bent and his purpose of sharing important lessons of historical change in Puerto Rico.

## *Memory Transfer*

Last, out of the three forms of mobilizations of memory explored in this section, what I call Memory Transfer is probably the most basic operation. It refers to the way that don José transferred his memories onto the wood while carving. This creative subprocess is also linked to the specificity of the medium. Don José told me that when he would work at his workshop in the *finca*, once a memory came to him, the process was simple as he had so many in mind. All that was miss-ing, he says, was more time: "The scene was easy to transfer into wood, because once I had the idea, that scene was already there and it simply would transfer. . . . [Sometimes] I carved pretty quickly . . . quite fast. . . . [I had] scenes on their way, on my mind; I had them, yes, so many of them, but I could not produce them all at once." As the above quote shows, after the other two operations, Identification and Compare and Contrast, were mobilized and the "right" internal image came to don José, carving was easy for him. This skill probably accounts for his prolific production of more than one hundred pieces created between the late 1970s and the 1980s. Don José carved until he could no longer accomplish the task as old age settled in and his hands now shake too much. Yet his collection continued to serve a purpose expanding into the realm of heritage.

## An Evolving Environment of Heritage

My main aim here is to introduce and contextualize from an on-the-ground perspective those main social actors, institutions, and other elements that have played a role and continue to do so in maintaining the "environment" of don José's woodcarvings as heritage.[19]

As don José stated, his late wife, doña Delia, played the key role in shaping this collection and was pivotal in safeguarding it: "There was a permanent place for them at home . . . a glass shelf [in the living room]. Delia would classify them.

. . . I received the stimulus of my wife, who enjoyed evaluating each piece and assigning it a place in the collection." It was in this space, originally in the urban house in which they lived before retiring, that the pieces found their first "soil." Then, when the couple retired, the collection was "transplanted" to their *finca*, finding its second "ground." The collection also grew during this time and doña Delia kept classifying and giving each piece value.

The curated pieces always attracted guests and other visitors, an audience— another important element—that contributed to the art's appreciation. In fact, don José even exhibited them twice in the capital San Juan, giving a conference presentation on one of these occasions. He says audiences responded well to his talks and his collection; some even wanted to buy pieces, and a number of people even visited his house to see it.

In 2005—five years before don José and doña Delia migrated to the United States—the collection was sent by mail northward to Christiansburg. There, in the Badillos' room by the main entrance underneath a loft, it was labeled and it found a curatorial niche.[20]

In Virginia, the pieces have also been exhibited beyond the home and to larger publics: once at the Montgomery Museum and Lewis Miller Regional Art Center, and then on a different occasion, the Christiansburg Recreation Center organized a field trip to the Badillo house for people see the sculptures and meet the artist. It was open to the public, and some of Sonia's students from her senior aerobics class seized the opportunity to learn firsthand. For this occasion, don José, with the help of Sonia, created an introductory text to help him tell his story and that of the collection.

But it is in the home environment, I argue, where those closest to don José have collectively given his woodcarvings value. For instance, I had the pleasure of meeting two of Sonia's grandchildren, five-year-old Ella and her two-and-a-half-year-old sister Evie. One afternoon, I witnessed Ella's interaction with the collection as well as with her little sister and grandmother in that space. Ella saw me taking photographs of each individual piece, and curiosity getting the best of her, she approached me and asked what I was doing. I explained, and then she shared with me her favorite figurines. "This one with the two girls is my favorite," she said. Why? Because they look so pretty (figs. 3.8 and 3.9). Moments later, Sonia joined us in the room and started to show little Ella and Evie some of the woodcarvings and explain to them the world that they conjure. A "little world" or "microcosm" that—contrary to don José's assertion that "time and succinct reality have taken care of . . . transforming into blurry shadows"—actually is re-created every time a wooden piece is picked up and knowledge about it passed on to new generations (figs. 3.10 and 3.11).

Such is the current "climate" and "soil type" of don José's woodcarvings as heritage. This environment has also been favored by other family members such

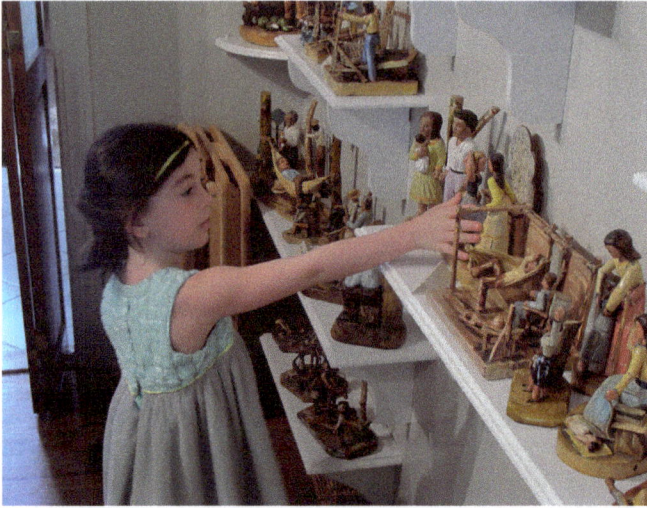

Fig. 3.8. Ella shows the author one of her favorite carvings, 2017. *Photograph by Julián Antonio Carrillo.*

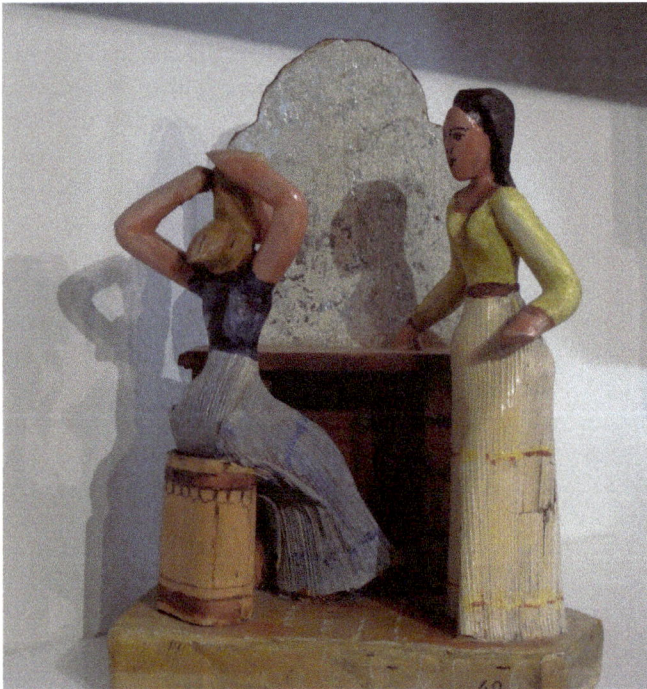

Fig. 3.9. "Two young women preparing for a fiesta," 2017. *Photograph by Julián Antonio Carrillo.*

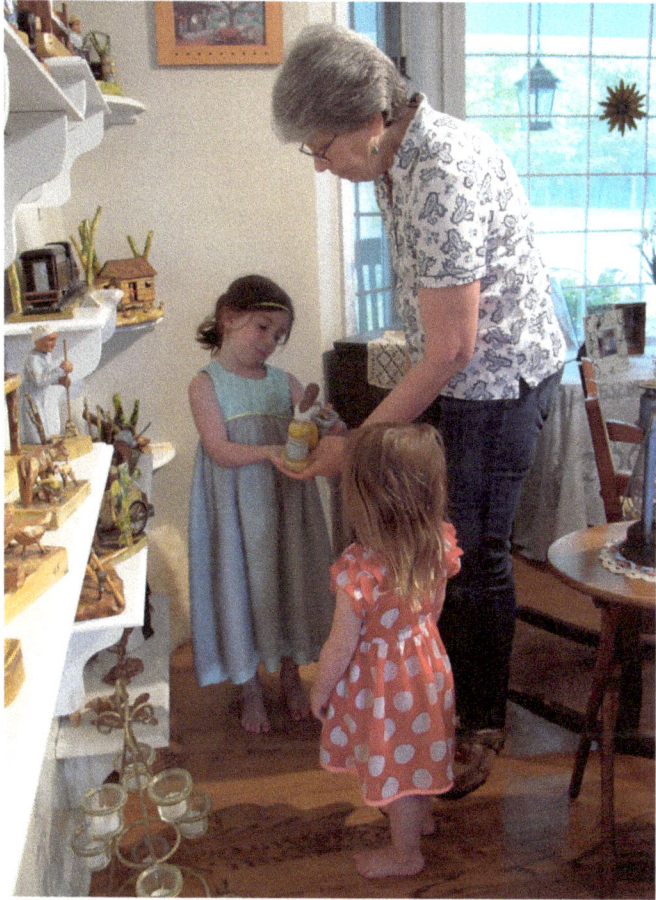

Fig. 3.10. Sonia showing her granddaughters select pieces, 2017. *Photograph by Julián Antonio Carrillo.*

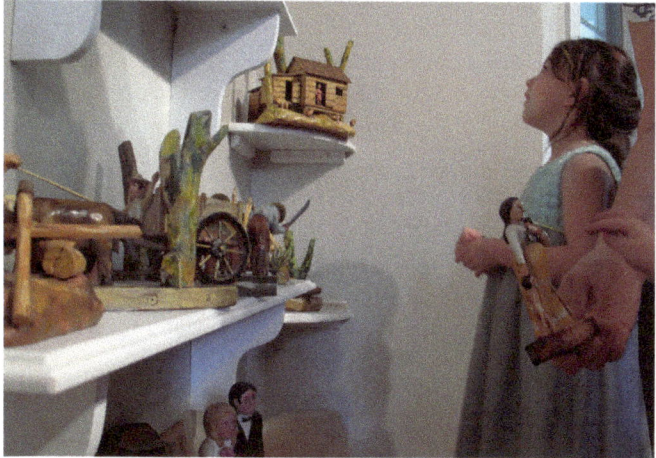

Fig. 3.11. Sonia telling her granddaughters about the pieces, 2017. *Photograph by Julián Antonio Carrillo.*

as Alex Badillo, whose "appreciation of the wooden sculptures as art and as an important historical depiction . . . has brought him to talk to others in his field and share 3-D pictures of them," as his mother Sonia puts it. In keeping with the environment metaphor, we can argue that Alex has "transplanted" the collection to a fourth new "ground," the virtual, with his photography.[21] Sonia further elaborates: "He has always felt that they were important and has worked at trying to expand their reach beyond our home and friends. We feel that it is thanks to his efforts that the connection was made with you [Julián] as a professional that could expose them and in turn many other connections are being made, too."

Indeed, Alex has acted as a mediator between the personal home environment and the wider spaces and places beyond it by inviting people like myself. I, too, hope to have played a role in the valorization of don José's woodcarving. Certainly, this chapter is thus far the clearest example, but leading up to its publication, I also shared pictures and a few texts about the collection with friends, family, and colleagues in person and online.

My efforts have led to other connections that Sonia mentions. For instance, in September 2017, Professor Danille Christensen took her Virginia Polytechnic Institute and State University folklore class to the Badillo home. Her students reportedly had a great experience, and don José enjoyed their visit very much. This was, in part, thanks to Jon Kay, director of Traditional Arts Indiana, who introduced Danille and me over the summer, and in turn, I introduced Danille to the Badillos. Now, there is talk of a possible exhibit of "Expressions" at her university's art museum in the near future.

As trained professionals in the field of folklore, we "have come to understand that our work is not simply studying the 'folk' but collaborating with them" (Zeitlin 2000, 14). Our collaborations should include fostering the emerging and ever-shifting environment of our collaborators' heritage and their creativity. Because as don José's case suggests, it is not only the art itself *but also its environment of valorization* that contributes to his well-being and that of others. This has important implications for the so-called creative aging industry[22] as well.

As the creative aging industry continues to develop, folklorists through our commitment to cultural activism and cultural democracy (Zeitlin 2000, 4) can help democratize it. But we also have something to offer elders by highlighting and working from the intra- and intergenerational connections that are crucial to the valorization of their folk arts as heritage. I suggest that bridging the private and public spheres, we propose ways to invite elder community scholars, artists, and others to new platforms from which they can socially engage other elders as well as new generations while demonstrating their creative expression and even skills mastery by promoting their own heritage and art.

## Conclusion

In this chapter, I presented a life history of Puerto Rican artist don José Lugo Arroyo and, characterizing his collection of woodcarvings as ethnographic, labeled him an ethnographic fieldworker. I focused on his creative process of woodcarving as I argue that it exhibits important dynamics and processes—what I referred to as "mobilizations of memory." I also focused on his folk art as heritage, introducing social actors and institutions that have worked to create and sustain its environment. In this last regard, I have argued that as folklorists, we can benefit our collaborators, audiences, and the emerging creative aging industry by focusing on and fostering the intra- and intergenerational ties on which such an environment of heritage is built and thrives.

Naturally, don José's life review period has not ended and he continues to reflect on every stage in his life. Attesting to this is his creative work that he does now. No longer being able to carve at ninety-three years, he still creates poetry and narratives on his computer. Not long ago, he finished and self-published his first novel, *Transculturation.* Currently, he is almost done with his latest project, *A Book for Those Who Have Nothing to Do.* It is a mixture of old and new poems, introspective narratives, and fun facts about the world, science, and history, meant to provide wonder and fulfillment to those who, perhaps like him, have "nothing" else to do in old age.

Yet, as I attempted to show, even though don José can no longer carve, the environment of appreciation of his woodcarvings live on years after he produced the last one. This environment, moreover, contributes not only to his well-being and health but also to that of his relatives, friends, and others. He is a source of pride, a role model, and an inspiration to many. The fact that don José is still creating at this late stage, even under deteriorating health conditions, is a testament to his convictions as well as to the power of art and expression. We, too, would be wise to value his art and that of many other older artists among us.

Julián Antonio Carrillo is a doctoral candidate in the Department of Anthropology at Indiana University.

## Works Cited

Emerson, Robert M., Rachel I. Fretz, and Linda L. Shaw. 1995. *Writing Ethnographic Fieldnotes.* Chicago: University of Chicago Press.

Foster, Michael Dylan, and Lisa Gilman. 2015. *UNESCO on the Ground: Local Perspectives on Intangible Cultural Heritage.* Bloomington: Indiana University Press.

Kay, Jon. 2016. *Folk Art and Aging.* Bloomington: Indiana University Press.

Kirshenblatt-Gimblett, Barbara. 1985. "Objects of Memory: Material Culture as Life Review." In *Folk Groups and Folklore Genres: A Reader*, edited by Elliott Oring, 329–38. Logan: Utah State University Press.

Mintz, Sidney. 1974. *Worker in the Cane: A Puerto Rican Life History*. New York: Norton.

Nash, June. 2005. "Defying Deterritorialization: Autonomy Movements against Globalization." In *Social Movements: An Anthropological Reader*, edited by June Nash, 177–86. Malden, MA: Blackwell.

Vogt, Wendy A. 2006. "Tracing Neoliberalism in Mexico: Historical Displacement and Survival Strategies for Mixtec Families Living on the U.S.-Mexico Border." MA thesis, University of Arizona, Tucson.

Zeitlin, Steven J. 2000. "I'm a Folklorist and You're Not: Expansive versus Delimited Strategies in the Practice of Folklore." *The Journal of American Folklore* 113 (447): 3–19.

## Notes

1. "Jibaro," *Merriam-Webster*, https://www.merriam-webster.com/dictionary/jibaro.

2. This Spanish word literally translates as "co-lived (with)," but its meaning is closer to "interacted (with)." *Convivir* is a type of meaningful interaction that leaves two or more people with a sense of having understood each other better. In this sense, it has a positive value. I spent from June 8–16, 2017, with don José and part of his family and have kept in touch ever since. During our *convivencia*, in addition to interviewing him and learning about his art, we bonded in discussing politics, sharing anecdotes, joking, cooking, eating, reading some of his poems aloud together, and even playing my songs on his old guitar for him. I thank him wholeheartedly for the time and opportunity to get to know each other.

3. The terms *don* for men and *doña* for women is used to respectfully address older people.

4. The term *figurine* might seem appropriate as it is "a statuette, especially one of a human form" (*New Oxford American Dictionary*). However, don José actually refers to his carvings as *estampas*, which means in Spanish a "figure or aspect of a person, animal, or object that produces a determined impression on a person who sees it" (my translation), according to the definition I found on Google (https://www.google.com/search?q=definicion+estampa&oq=definicion+estampa&aqs=chrome..69i57.4825j0j8&sourceid=chrome&ie=UTF-8). In this chapter, I use the words *figurines*, *carvings*, and other terms interchangeably to refer to his collection.

5. Steve Zeitlin argues that historically folklorists have taken both delimiting and expansive approaches to defining what counts as folklore as well as who counts as a folklorist, employing these approaches strategically depending on time and place (Zeitlin 2000, 3): "The delimited stance carefully defines and limits the discipline, studies its own history, strives for professionalization, and creates a justification for an autonomous field. The expansive posture, on the other hand, tries to establish alliances and explores other disciplines freely, asserting that other arts and humanities fields have as much right to practice folklore as folklorists have to practice those fields. Expansive positions often reach out to new members, constituencies, and audiences."

In this chapter, I adopt a decidedly expansive approach by strategically treating don José as a folkloristic "ethnographic fieldworker" and his carvings as a folkloristic "ethnographic" collection. His grandson and archaeologist Alex E. Badillo has referred to the woodcarvings as "ethnographic scenes." Here, I take this further, arguing that not only is his collection constituted by ethnographic scenes but also that don José can be rightly called an "ethnographic fieldworker." Emerson, Fretz, and Shaw (1995, 1) state that

> ethnographic field research involves the study of groups and people as they go about their everyday lives. Carrying out such research involves two distinct activities. First, the ethnographer enters into a social setting and gets to know the people involved in it; usually, the setting is not previously known in an intimate way. The ethnographer participates in the daily routines of this setting, develops ongoing relations with the people in it, and observes all the while what is going on. Indeed, the term "participant observation" is often used to characterize this basic research approach. But, second, the ethnographer writes down in regular, systematic ways what she observes and learns while participating in the daily rounds of life of others. Thus the researcher creates an accumulating written record of these observations and experiences. These two interconnected activities comprise the core of ethnographic research: Firsthand participation in some initially unfamiliar social world and the production of written accounts of that world by drawing upon such participation.

My intention in calling don José a folkloristic "ethnographer" and his artwork "ethnographic" is not to discredit colleagues who have conducted professional ethnographies nor undermine those who have studied folkloristics academically and conduct field research in this field. Don José certainly did not undertake a great deal of what is involved in "writing ethnographic field notes" (Emerson, Fretz, and Shaw 1995).

However, as I hope this chapter demonstrates, don José participated in the daily routines of his neighborhood and village in rural Puerto Rico, getting to know the people involved in this setting in both intimate and non-intimate ways and observing "all" that was going on. Moreover, don José inscribed in his memory what he observed and learned while participating in the daily rounds of the lives of others. As later sections of the chapter will make clear, don José also carved his observations beginning in his youth, which helped him develop muscle memory that he would draw on in his adult years when he created an accumulating *carved* record of these experiences that would become his collection. Last, his carved, permanent material record of memories enables his *spoken* and *embodied* record of observations and experiences to be shared with others, like myself during interviews or like newer generations of his family.

6. Alex Badillo told me about his grandfather's figures and said he was looking for someone to interview him. As a folkloristic anthropologist with an interest in the heritage of Latinos, Latin America, and the Caribbean, I was drawn to his carvings and wanted to know more about them and their value. Soon after this initial conversation, Alex spoke to his parents and put them in touch with me. A few weeks later, in June 2017, I paid them a visit in Virginia. I am grateful for their warm welcome in their home and for taking time from their busy schedule. I would also like to thank Alex, of course, who made it all possible. In addition, I would like to thank Jon Kay, Isis Sadek, Elena Papadakos, Matthew Lebrato, Danille Christensen, and two anonymous reviewers for their feedback on drafts of this chapter.

7. All conversations and interviews with don José were in Spanish. I translated them for this chapter.

8. While the word *parranda* can refer to any gathering or party, those that occur in Puerto Rico during the Christmas season, which spans past December 25 into January 6 when the Feast of Epiphany is celebrated, consist of serenading friends and relatives with festive music during the night.

9. A musical genre in Puerto Rico and other places with Hispanic cultural influence commonly performed during the Christmas season, lyrics can be religious or secular.

10. Similar to Vogt's (2006, 30) and Nash's (2005, 178) perspectives, I view modernization, migration, deterritorialization, displacement, and, I would add, "professionalization," among others, as inseparable from and connected to the processes of capitalism, not as processes in themselves.

11. As further evidence of don José's ethnographic inclination not only in carving but also in the stories he shares, when he explained to me the *"parranda"* figure mentioned above, he said that today this *viejísima* (extremely old) tradition is no longer practiced in the same way. Whereas before it took place in his family and inside homes, today, he says, the *velorio* (a nocturnal social gathering featuring dances, singing, and stories, and celebrated in the houses of small towns) is held in the town hall where locals go to sing songs and play music. As such, he was documenting for posterity a changing or dying tradition.

12. The condensed life history I provide in the next section is largely based on a 2005 autobiographical text in Spanish called, "Box of Memories," which, as stated on p. 77, "is a product of joint efforts of both of us [don José and doña Delia], as everything else has been in our lives." In translating excerpts from this text, I respect his/their original wording as much as possible and if I leave out some important things, it is only because of limited time and space.

13. A blessing, made with the sign of the cross over (*Oxford Spanish Dictionary*, 3rd ed.).

14. A kind of gramophone used particularly in the 1920s and 1930s.

15. While this life review continued even after don José and doña Delia left Puerto Rico to live in the United States, and even continues today as don José still makes other types of art (poetry, fiction, and nonfiction), the production of the one hundred wooden memory objects marks its intense beginning and is thus worthy of our attention.

16. I decided to keep the original Spanish word, as *pueblo* means both "people" and "town," and he used the term in a way that could refer to both.

17. For example, consider the figurine of the "Boy milking a cow." In an interview, he confirmed that this piece, which not coincidentally was the first one he carved during his life review period that became a permanent part of the collection, was not the first woodcarving of this memory that he had made. He had made others, since he was a boy, but had always thrown them away not seeing more value in them than the mere enjoyment of the process of making them. This shows us that sometimes timing is everything, and indeed life review is a powerful period in the expressive lives of elders.

18. This quote also comes from the aforementioned "Box of Memories," of which this map is a part. In translating his quotes, I have respected don José's words as much as possible, yet in a few cases in which he originally wrote in the third person, my translations have used the first person in order to make the reading more fluid. For example, where he wrote, "data that resides in the memory of the author," I changed to, "data that resides in my memory."

19. Michael Foster argues that an on-the-ground perspective to heritage and heritage making that wants to avoid "missing the trees for the forest," requires an "effort to burrow into the foliage of particular cultures, communities, and places to discover the trees themselves" (Foster and Gilman 2015, 4). What we learn through this process, he continues, "is that different forests are constituted in different ways, that not all trees are equal, and that not all trees have the same relationship to the forest in which they are located. To extend the metaphor even further, what is driven home to us along with the diversity of individual trees is the *range of soils and climates and the many other elements that create the environment in which they grow*" (Foster and Gilman 2015, 4, emphasis added).

20. Sonia Badillo grouped the objects in the collection by themes thought out by her former daughter-in-law, Niki Dula.

21. For six of these models and more, please visit Alex's Sketchfab page: https://skfb.ly /6uABs.

22. The website creativeagingtoolkit.org defines creative aging as "the practice of engaging older adults (55+) in participatory, professionally run arts programs with a focus on social engagement and skills mastery. This movement is about providing opportunity for meaningful creative expression through visual, literary, and performing arts workshops."

# 4  The Role of Traditional Arts in Identity Creation in the Lives of Elders

Patricia A. Atkinson

In a small workshop behind his house, a slim ninety-eight-year-old man is busy working with wood, deer antler, and stone. He is sculpting, sanding, and polishing these materials to make a ceremonial pipe. His workshop is full of tools of all sizes, reflective of his work life as a master carpenter as well as his interest in shaping stones to create pipe bowls (fig. 4.1). His apprentice, a man in his fifties, has tightened an emerging stone bowl into a vise and is using a rasp and file to shape the stone. The elder is delighted to show off his workshop, his tools, his materials, and his finished pipes. These are labor-intensive pieces and regarded by many as works of art. He does not sell his pipes, although he has had many offers. He regards them as sacred objects to be used for prayer, not art pieces for display. He gives them to those he deems worthy—or in need of spiritual guidance or cleansing—as ceremonial tools used to send prayers to Creator. He is proud to be known as a pipe maker, not only to his family and immediate community but also to the larger community of Paiute, Washoe, and Shoshone people of the Great Basin as well as native people from other parts of the United States and the world. While pipe making is not a tradition native to the Northern Paiute tribe into which he was born, the adoption and use of ceremonial pipes by northern Nevada's indigenous people dates back more than sixty years. Following World War II, the Bureau of Indian Affairs instituted an urbanization program that sent members of American Indian tribes to cities—many to the West Coast to Los Angeles and the San Francisco area. During this era, the people were introduced

*The Expressive Lives of Elders* (2018): 80–94, DOI: 10.2979/expressivelivesofelders.0.0.05

Fig. 4.1. The pipe maker in his workshop. *Photograph by Rebecca Snetselaar. Courtesy of the Nevada Folklife Archive, Nevada Arts Council.*

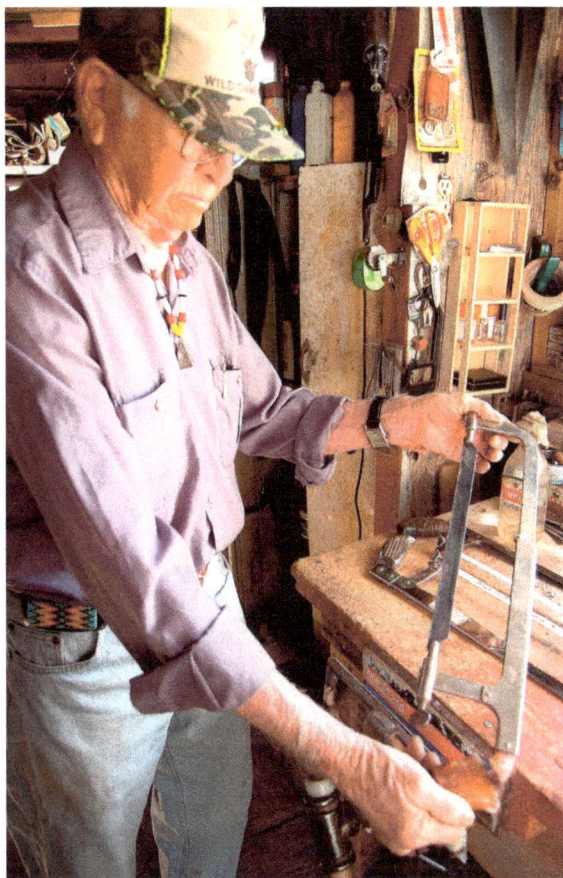

to each other's traditions and a number of Plains Indian traditions—including dance styles and ceremonial objects—were embraced by the Northern Paiutes.

As the director of a state public folklife program, one of my duties has been to administer an apprenticeship program in folk and traditional arts. During my decade in this position, I have become aware that the demographics of the master and apprentice pairs have changed from the standard model of an elder community member teaching a youthful apprentice. A number of apprentices have been middle-aged or elderly individuals; master artists may be teaching peers their own age or older members of their communities. I began to wonder about this phenomenon. What was going on here? Did these apprentices in different ethnic groups have anything in common other than their ages? Was there a significance to middle age and/or post-retirement?

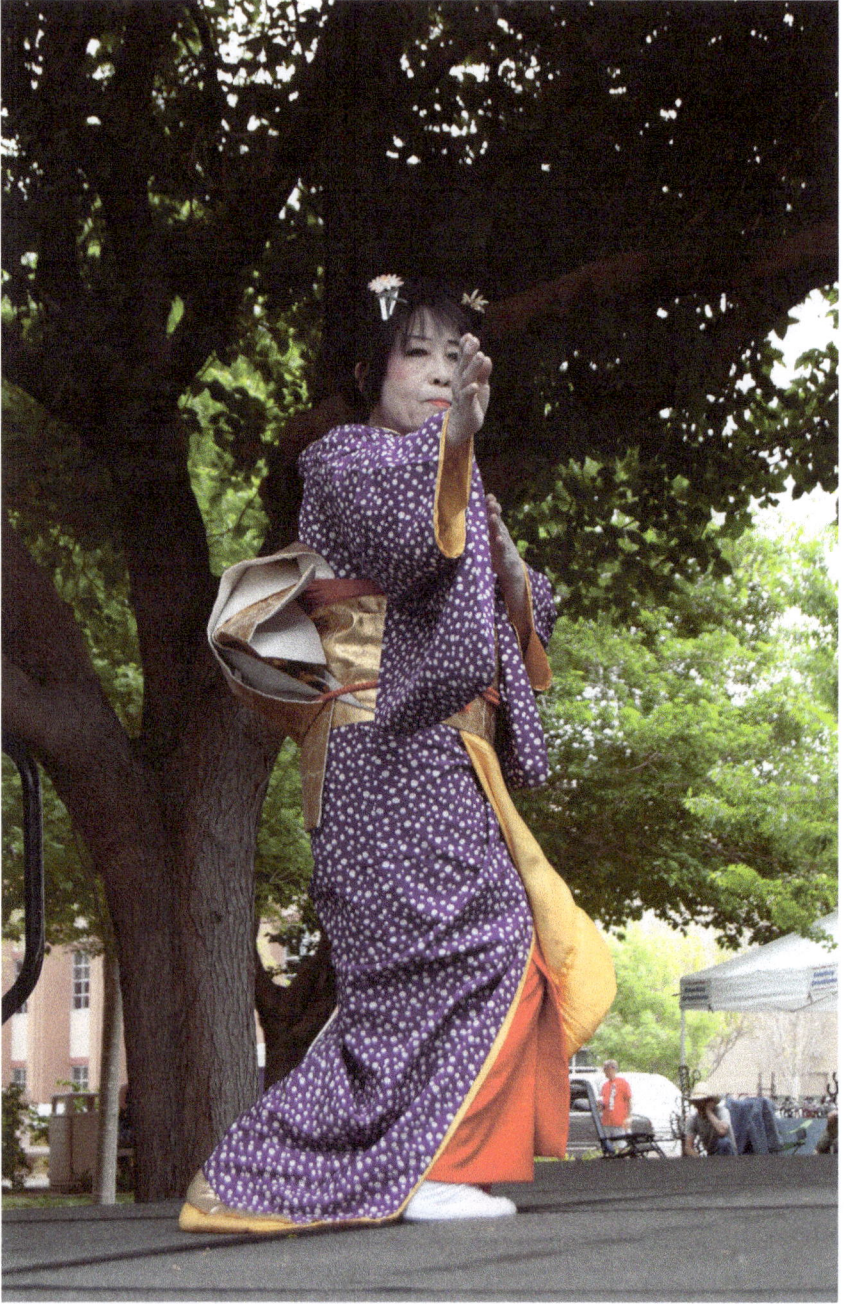

Fig. 4.2. Master dancer Fumiko Duncan. *Photograph by Rebecca Snetselaar. Courtesy of the Nevada Folklife Archives.*

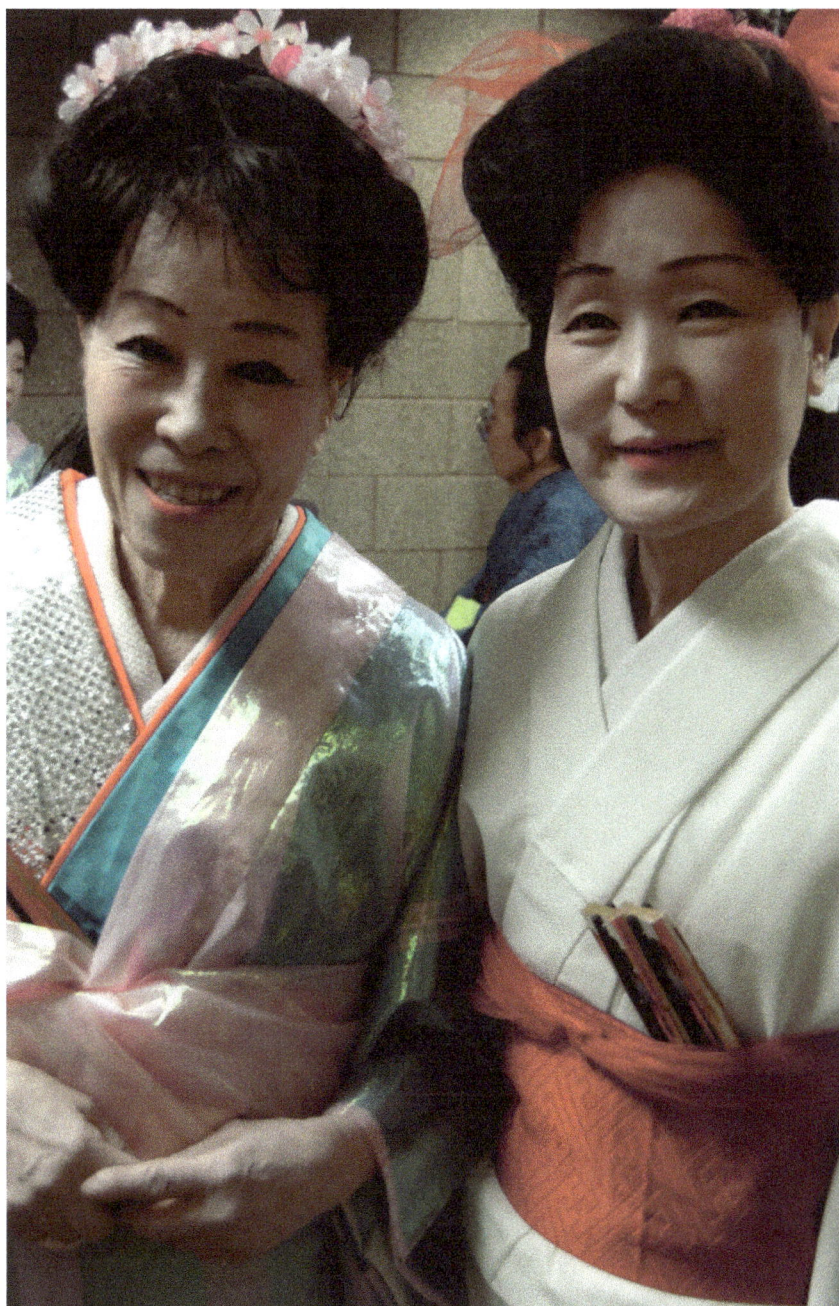

Fig. 4.3. Apprentice Christine Ohira (left) with master dancer Fumiko Duncan. *Photograph by Rebecca Snetselaar. Courtesy of the Nevada Folklife Archives.*

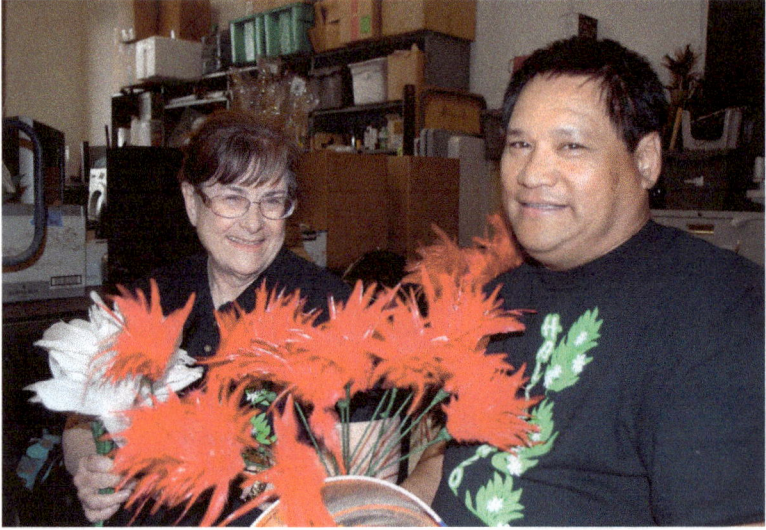

Fig. 4.4. Making feather kahili. Master artist Charles Herring and apprentice Patricia Gorsch. *Photograph by Rebecca Snetselaar. Courtesy of the Nevada Folklife Archives.*

My engagement with the master and apprentice artists in these "upside-down" apprenticeships is best comprehended by presenting their stories. While I will introduce the reader to several Nevada traditional artists, they are by no means the only examples of this phenomenon.

Once a week, forty-five weeks each year, for the last twelve years, Fumiko Duncan has taught traditional Japanese Tendo dance to groups of Japanese American women at the West Flamingo Senior Center in Las Vegas (fig. 4.2). Fumiko studied Tendo, a twentieth-century style of Kabuki, in her native Japan with Miyoko Maruyama, who created Tendo dance in the 1950s. Now in her senior years, Fumiko is a certified master instructor.

The senior women study and practice dance and the use of dance accessories such as fans, umbrellas, and flowers for two hours each week. They meet between August 1 and March 30 to prepare for performances as the Tendo Baikoki group, which performs at Chinese New Year, the Aki Matsuri Festival, the Martin Luther King Day parade, the Henderson Heritage Parade, and other community functions (fig. 4.3).

Hawaiian native Charles Herring, who lives in Las Vegas, holds regular hula classes for seniors and teaches lei making, palm frond basketry, and the crafting of feather leis and *kahili* to apprentices, some twenty to thirty years older than he is (fig. 4.4). Many Native Hawaiians and Hawaiian-born individuals have settled

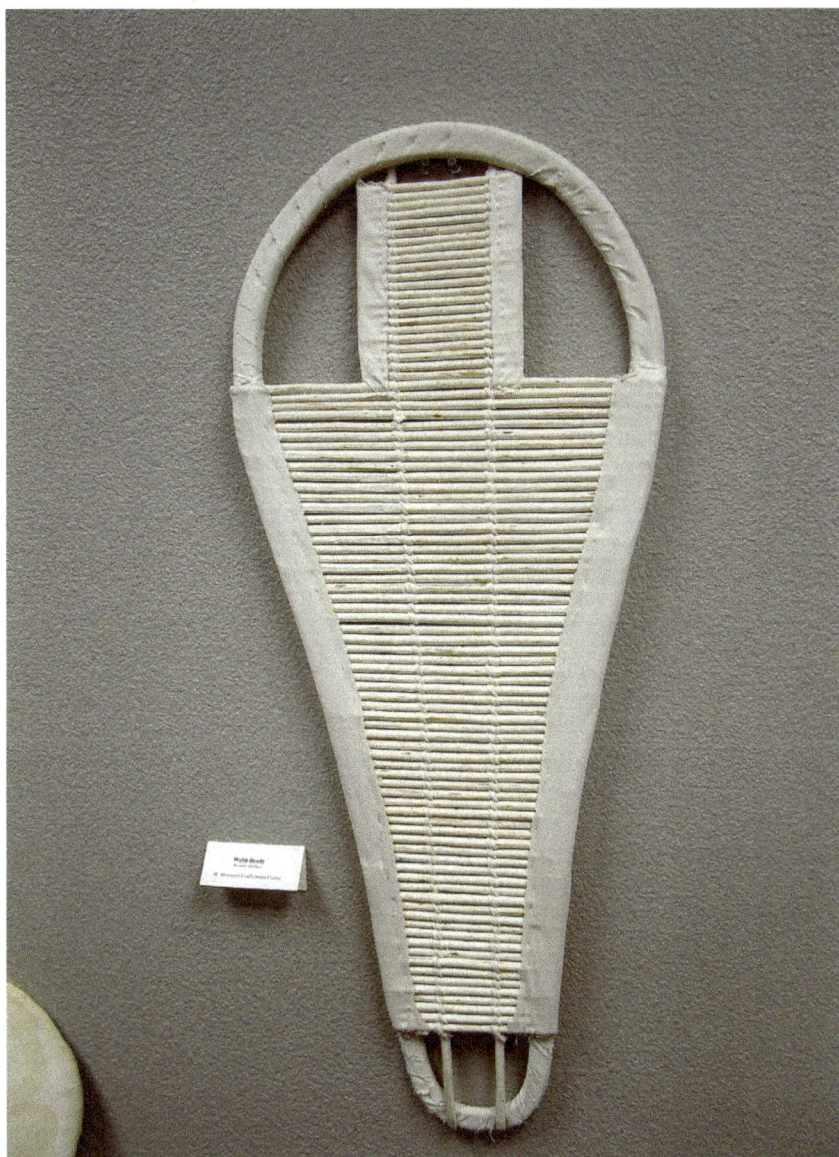

Fig. 4.5. Shoshone Cradleboard Frame. *Photograph by Patricia A. Atkinson. Courtesy of the Nevada Folklife Archives.*

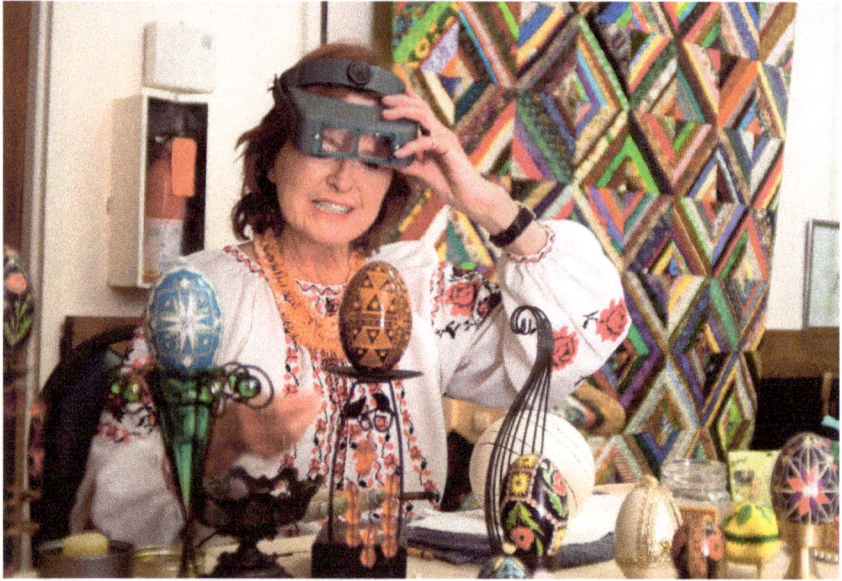

Fig. 4.6. Former apprentice, now master pysanky artist Joyce Brittan Kasady. *Photograph by Rebecca Snetselaar. Courtesy of the Nevada Folklife Archives.*

in Las Vegas and work to maintain and/or express Hawaiian identity through participation in traditional arts, foodways, and cultural festivals. Las Vegas is known to Hawaiians in the islands, as well as on the mainland, as the "Ninth Island" (the state of Hawaii comprises eight islands) because of the large population of Hawaiians who have settled in the Las Vegas area. This has mainly been due to the availability of jobs in hospitality and performing arts, which are deeply tied to the gaming industry and to the lower cost of living and real property in Nevada.

Shoshone master traditional artists Leah Brady and Roger Ike, both in their late-fifties/early sixties, regularly teach the arts of willow cradleboard making (fig. 4.5) and quilting to seniors in the local Shoshone-Paiute community and at the Duck Valley Reservation in Owyhee, Nevada, some ninety-seven miles from Elko. Also active in the Shoshone language revitalization movement, Brady and Ike are passing on traditional skills that they learned from elders in their families to age peers and seniors who did not have opportunities to learn when they were younger.

For several decades, until she was well into her nineties, Ukrainian *pysanky* master Zoria Zetaruk taught weekly classes in "egg writing" at a Las Vegas senior center. Many retirees of Ukrainian origin came to learn from Zoria, and two of

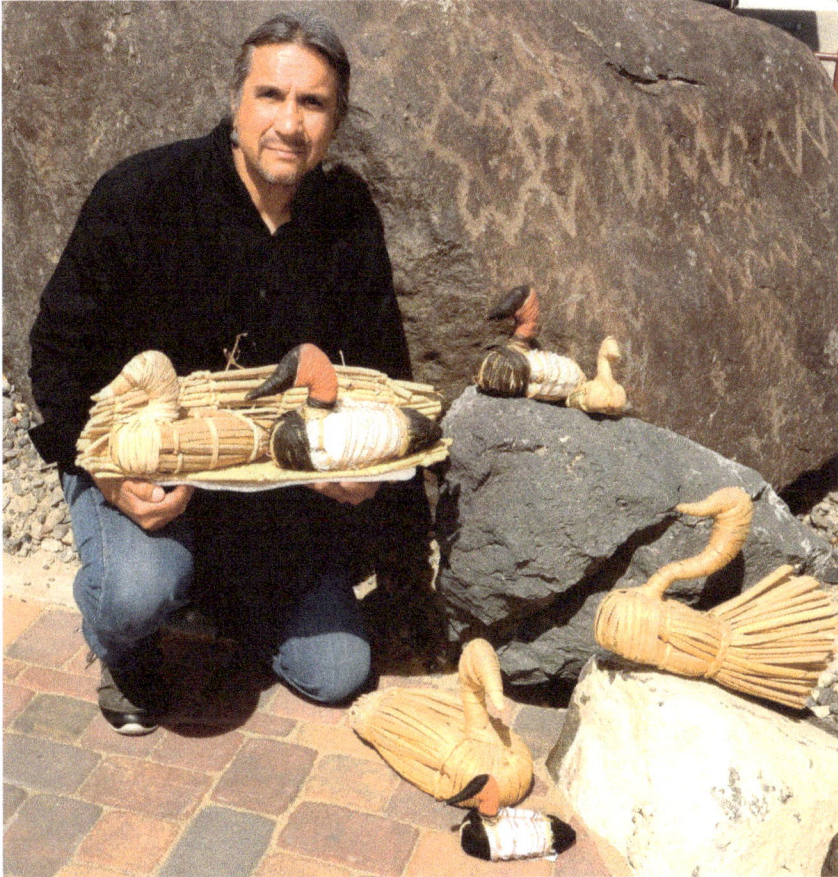

Fig. 4.7. Master Tule artist Mike Williams. *Photograph by Patricia A. Atkinson. Courtesy of the Nevada Folklife Archives.*

her senior apprentices became master teaching artists through the Nevada Arts Council's Folklife Apprenticeship Program as a way to continue connections to Ukrainian traditions in the desert and amid the neon (fig. 4.6).

A number of Nevada's twenty-six tribal entities have regular language and culture study groups—some specifically for seniors, others multigenerational—to try to preserve and perpetuate cultural knowledge in the face of the loss of tradition through government-mandated assimilation (Indian boarding schools and urbanization movements) and other policies that took tribal members away from their homelands and placed them in cities. The Pyramid Lake Paiute Tribe Museum regularly hosts workshops in such skills as basket weaving, beading, and buckskin work. Most of those who attend are between the ages of thirty-five and seventy-five.

Master traditional tule artist Mike Williams of Stillwater taught a two-day workshop at Pyramid Lake on the weaving of tule mats in conjunction with the repatriation of human remains stolen from a cave burial (fig. 4.7). The ancestors buried their dead in caves lying on tule mats, and the tribe wanted to honor the deceased by reinterring them in the most traditional way possible. The participants were primarily individuals in their fifties to seventies. Williams became conversant in traditional tule arts only after retirement, when he moved from Carson City to a reservation with marshlands near Fallon.

Why this upsurge in learning folk and traditional arts in midlife or post-retirement? When I asked Fumiko Duncan why the folk/traditional arts are important in the Japanese community in Las Vegas, I received the following answer:

> To be a "hyphenated American" is to have a foot in two cultures and to experience pressures to completely assimilate. For many seniors in the Japanese American community, this pressure has been negative, including cultural stereotypes and racially based discrimination. Japanese Americans are ethnically diverse, and our differences pose many questions. Many seniors never had the opportunity to learn Japanese cultural arts when they were younger. Experiencing traditional Japanese folk arts is a vital way to counter these negative messages, to develop an affirming sense of community and to build positive cultural identity in the senior students, who take pride in participating in public performances. Japanese traditional arts are meant to be performed at private family celebrations and in public. The seniors who belong to the Tendo Baikoki group have many opportunities to share what they have learned with their own families as well as in public performances and cultural displays at events, parades, schools, libraries, clubs, and churches.

For each of the artists I have introduced, cultural disruption or physical relocation is an important component in their life's journey. Cultural disruption in its most drastic and dramatic form took place for Nevada tribal members who were sent to boarding schools where they were either discouraged from or forbidden to engage in their languages and cultural practices. The generation that came after them was bereft of elders to teach them their traditions, and consequently a large proportion did not learn their tribes' traditional culture. Another segment of this group was sent to cities in their late teens or early twenties to become disenfranchised "urban Indians," assimilating completely and/or learning traditions of other tribes and adopting them as their own. Pan-Indian powwow outfits, dances, crafts, and foodways such as Indian tacos (seasoned ground meat, beans, cheese, and lettuce on fry bread) are interesting examples of adopted and adapted tribal traditions.

The young Japanese women who married Americans and were brought back to their husbands' home communities experienced familial and social pressure

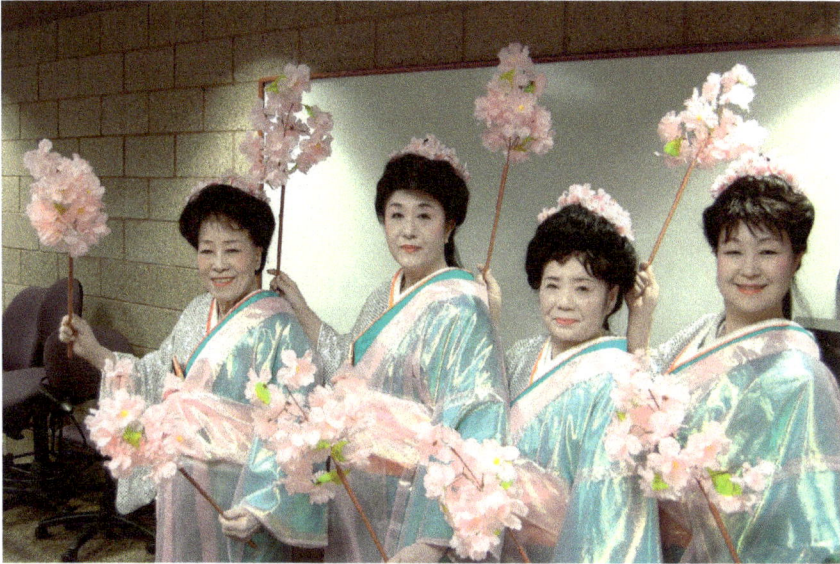

Fig. 4.8. Tendo Baikoki back stage. *Photograph by Rebecca Snetselaar. Courtesy of the Nevada Folklife Archives.*

to assimilate and to be "American" in their food, dress, and behavior. Fumiko Duncan talks about "having a foot in each culture" and describes the lack of ways to express and celebrate Japanese identity during the early years of marriage and motherhood. She draws attention to "affirming a sense of community" and "building a positive cultural identity" as fundamental motives for engaging in cultural practices viewed as traditional and expressive of a particular identity (fig. 4.8).

For the Hawaiian residents of the Ninth Island," the move from tropical islands to the open desert landscape of southern Nevada is a significant change and can be considered as both psychological and emotional disruption. As much of Hawaiian traditional culture evolved in and springs from the unique ecosystem of the islands, being separated from that environment means the absence of cultural landscape and materials necessary for traditional cultural expression. Businesses that import such supplies and restaurants that prepare traditional Hawaiian foods thrive in Las Vegas.

In his essay "'Tradition' in Identity Discourses and an Individual's Symbolic Construction of Self," Michael Owen Jones (2000, 115–41) presents a close study of an individual who "chooses from tradition those behaviors, activities and objects with which he can symbolically construct an identity." He cites a number of scholarly works that have examined the relationship between identity and tradition, including those that focus on individuals and others that are concerned with group practices and collective cultural identity. In the conclusion to his essay, Jones (2000, 134) states that "individuals often self-consciously adopt and adapt tradition as an element in their discourse about who they are or want to be, utilizing tradition in the symbolic construction of their identity. This indicates that a direction for future research is to explore explicitly the processes of choosing from tradition in order to symbolically construct an identity, and to examine in greater detail the motivations for and means of doing so."

In "The Arts, Artifacts, and Artifices of Identity," Elliott Oring (1994, 223) asserts that humans have "sense of identity rooted in artistic production" and that "when we define and redefine folklore, we are conceptualizing and reconceptualizing a set of cultural materials and their privileged relation to the identities of individuals and groups." Engagement with traditional arts "serves to enhance efforts to delineate personal and cultural identity" (Oring 1994, 222).

Jon Kay is one of a new generation of folklorists who are examining the creative lives of older adults. In his book *Folk Art and Aging: Life-Story Objects and Their Makers*, Kay (2016) introduces five elders who are connecting with others and forging new identities in their later years. In particular, Kay looks at the relationships between individuals, their art, their narrations about their lives triggered by presenting their art, and the performance of identity that occurs in these narrations. Troyd Geist's (2017) significant work with North Dakota's Art for Life Program for Elders has taken him from the familiar realms of traditional art into gerontology and neuroscience while examining significance of nostalgia and life review.

While standing on the shoulders of these scholars, I have approached traditional arts among elders from a somewhat different direction, taking to heart Michael Owen Jones's (2000, 134) directive "to explore explicitly the processes of choosing from tradition in order to symbolically construct an identity, and to examine in greater detail the motivations for and means of doing so."

The theme of the conference for which this essay was first envisioned—Resistance, Reclamation, and Re-creation—applies well to aging individuals. Those who are nearing retirement age—or past retirement age—will be familiar with the reams of material aimed at seniors regarding loss of bodily functions, loss of job-based identity, loss of mobility, and so forth. Many elders resist these marketing stereotypes and reclaim an identity as part of a traditional group; others invent new identities as creative individuals—as we have seen in Jon Kay's work with elders and life-story objects.

Some older adults may re-create or recover a cultural identity that they feel was lost due to cultural disruption through some kind of displacement or disconnection from their cultural group, homeland, community, language, and so on. When their time becomes their own, or when they are engaged in life re-

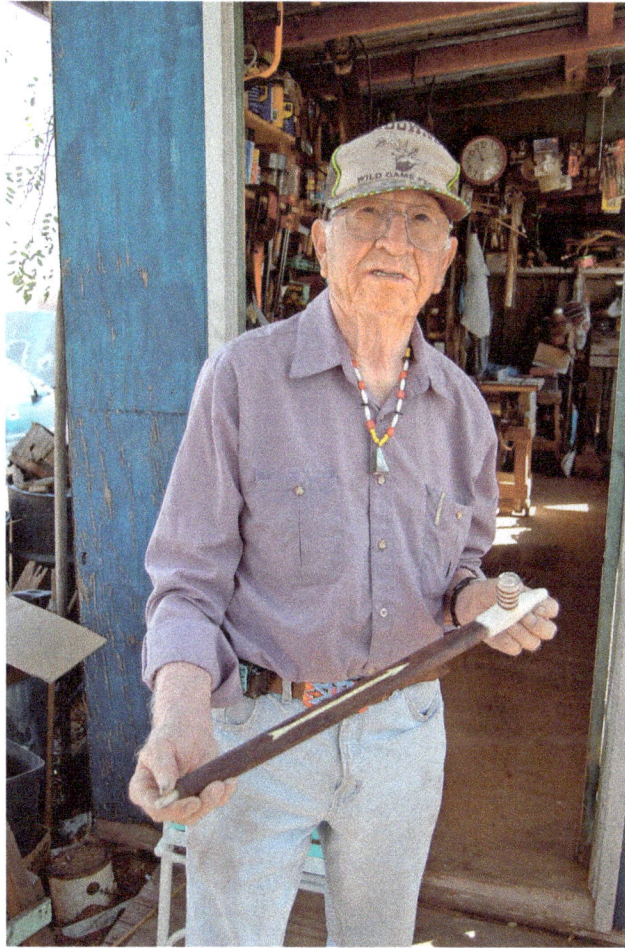

Fig. 4.9. Hilman Tobey, master pipe maker. *Photograph by Gabe Lopez Shaw. Courtesy of the Nevada Folklife Archives.*

view, they actively engage in the traditions of their families or communities as a way to reassert or reclaim a cultural identity. While I initially thought of this as "reconnection," thanks to Troyd Geist's study of creativity and neuroscience, I now understand this as making new connections—both new neural connections, which help to regenerate the brain, and new community/family/group connections, which remind us that "traditions are symbolic constructions of the past in the present for the future" (Jones 2000, 116).

I'd like to present one more example of an apprenticeship—this one was not upside-down but featured the master traditional artist and apprentice I described in the opening of this chapter. Hilman Tobey was born to the Pyramid Lake Pai-

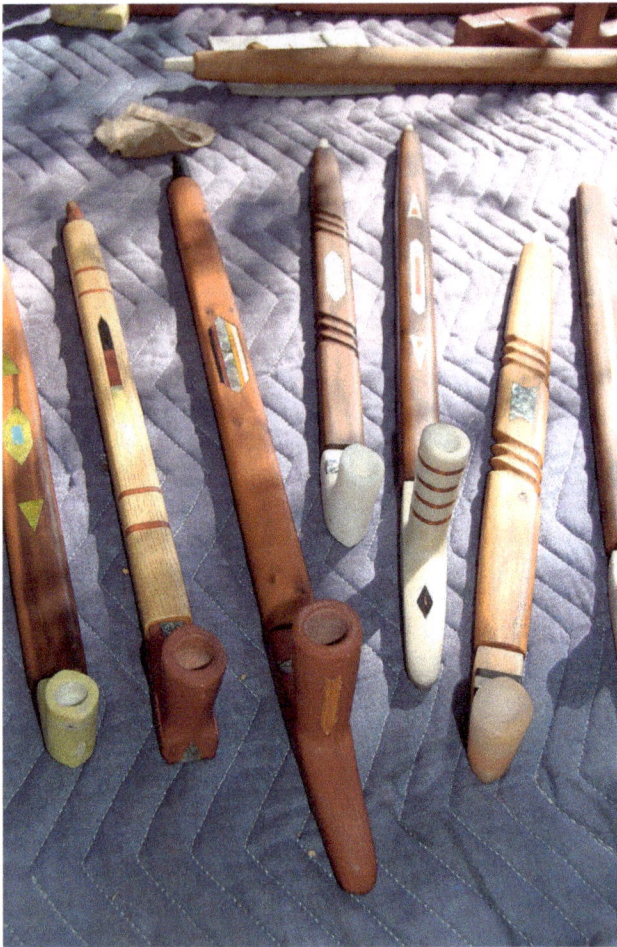

Fig. 4.10. Pipes by Hilman Tobey. *Photograph by Rebecca Snetselaar. Courtesy of the Nevada Folklife Archives.*

ute Tribe in 1915 and was sent to the Stewart Indian School at the age of eleven, speaking only Paiute. At Stewart, he learned to speak and read English and studied mechanical drawing and carpentry. After graduating, Hilman worked with the Civilian Conservation Corps in the forests of eastern Oregon near the Warm Springs Reservation, where he cleared roads and learned surveying. From there, he worked as a surveyor for irrigation projects, then went to Hawthorne, Nevada, where he helped build ammunition storage depots and bunkers. Moving to Riverside, California, he worked for a company that built equipment for the fruit-packing industry. The company secured a draft deferment for him as his job was deemed essential to the war effort. In 1947, he became a member of the carpenters union (Nevada Arts Council 2015).[1]

After the war, Hilman moved to the Reno-Sparks Indian Colony and bought the lot next to where his brother resided. He worked in civilian construction and carpentry in Nevada until his retirement in 1980. He was very proud of his sixty-seven-year membership in Reno Carpenters Local Union 971. During his thirty-six years of retirement, he became interested in stonework and began making ceremonial pipes (fig. 4.9). This turned out to be an important aspect of his post-retirement identity—he became known as the pipe maker. As part of the documentation of the apprenticeship, I commissioned a Paiute filmmaker to record and present Hilman in his workshop—at age ninety-eight—with apprentice Norman, then in his early fifties. Both men emphasized the spiritual nature of their work and the importance of "thinking right" and "doing right" when making and using ceremonial pipes. Although the tradition of ceremonial pipes did not originate with the Northern Paiutes, it has been adopted as an important feature of spiritual practices such as those that take place in the sweat lodge. Čhaŋnúŋpa (in Standard Lakota Orthography) is the Sioux language name for the sacred ceremonial pipe and the ceremony in which it is used. "Pipe maker" was how Hilman chose to identify himself in later life. Norman, in middle age, was putting his life back together following some personal challenges. Returning to the reservation and taking up a traditional art form with a respected elder allowed Norman to begin to adopt a new and respectable identity, both within and outside his traditional group (fig. 4.10).

Why are a reconnection with tradition and the assertion of a creative and/ or cultural identity important? Elders are metaphorically drowning in a sea of negative messages about aging. Connections with traditions and creative endeavors are life affirming, they are positive. They create connections in the brain and within families and communities. For people who have suffered a loss of tradition, language, or community, a return to the familiarity of traditional lifeways helps to create or restore balance in lives marked by chaos. In these days of digital media, virtual reality, and increased isolation, participation in the traditional arts may be what keeps people engaged with their families, their communities, and the world around them. This has implications for those who work with older adults, for people working in refugee resettlement and with other types of immigrant communities, and for public folklorists in grant-making programs. Support for the preservation and perpetuation of folk and traditional arts can help stabilize communities and contribute to both mental and physical health and wellness.

Patricia Atkinson is Folklife Director at the Nevada Arts Council. She has authored the *Handbook for Folk and Traditional Artists* for the states of Tennessee, Nevada, and North Carolina and serves on the board of the American Folklife Center at the Library of Congress.

## Works Cited

Geist, Troyd. 2017. *Sundogs and Sunflowers: An Art for Life Program Guide for Creative Aging, Health and Wellness*. Bismarck: North Dakota Council on the Arts.

Jones, Michael Owen. 2000. "'Tradition" in Identity Discourses and an Individual's Symbolic Construction of Self." *Western Folklore* 59: 115–40.

Kay, Jon. 2016. *Folk Art and Aging: Life-Story Objects and Their Makers*. Bloomington: Indiana University Press.

Nevada Arts Council. 2015. *Nevada Stories: Pipe Makers of the Great Basin*. Filmed by Gabe Lopez Shaw for the Folklife Program of the Nevada Arts Council. Carson City: Nevada Arts Council.

Oring, Elliott. 1994. "The Arts, Artifacts, and Artifices of Identity." *Journal of American Folklore* 107 (242): 211–33. http://www.jstor.org/stable/541199.

## Notes

1. Hilman Tobey, oral history interview with Terry McBride for the Reno-Sparks Indian Colony Cultural Resources Program, 2005. Thanks to Michon R. Eben, tribal historic preservation officer, and Allan Tobey, program assistant/oral historian.

# 5   "I Don't Have Time to Be Bored"

## Creativity of a Senior Weaver

### Yvonne R. Lockwood

THROUGHOUT THE HISTORY of folklore studies, elderly tradition bearers have been an important resource as the maintainers of cultural knowledge and tradition. However, only recently have researchers begun to examine how folk traditions can play an important part in making one's senior years a positive experience and helped to change the prevailing negative view of aging. (See, for example, Hufford, Hunt, and Zeitlin 1987; Schuldiner 1994; Kay 2016.)

In addressing the theme of aging and creativity, I review the life and creative expressions of Anna Lassila, a master craftsperson whose primary artistic outlet was rag rug weaving. Although she enthusiastically and skillfully engaged in Finnish folk traditions most of her adult life, there was a notable change in self-awareness when she was in her eighties.

Of the thousands of immigrants from Europe between 1880 and 1920 with knowledge of rag rug weaving, Finns have maintained it best. Finns have woven rag rugs since before emigration from Finland. The continuity of this tradition can be attributed to Finnish American ethnicity; rag rugs and rug weaving are iconic ethnic folk traditions (Lockwood 2010). Anna was one of the many weavers interviewed in the 1980s and 1990s in a major research project about Finnish American rag rugs and weavers (Lockwood 2010, 32–44).[1]

An immigrant's life in Michigan's Upper Peninsula in the first decades of the twentieth century was not easy. Men commonly worked in the woods or mines, while the women and children worked the subsistence farm, if they were lucky to own land that had been cleared of huge boulders and thick woods.[2] This was the context in which Anna, a first-generation Finnish American, lived. Born in

*The Expressive Lives of Elders* (2018): 95–105, DOI: 10.2979/expressivelivesofelders.0.0.06

1909, a year after her parents arrived in the United States, and the oldest of eight siblings, Anna had a heavy load of responsibilities. Out of absolute necessity, she learned all the domestic skills—baking, cooking, food preservation, soap making, sewing, knitting, crocheting, feather pillow making, and even woodworking. Working alongside her mother, she was responsible for household duties and caring for her younger siblings. At thirteen, she was sewing clothes for her siblings and learned to weave from a neighbor farm wife.

An important fact about Anna is her faith, which explains her worldview, core values, and even her perpetuation of Finnish American tradition. Anna was Apostolic (or Laestadian), a strict form of Lutheranism that does not allow dancing, makeup, short hair for women, short skirts, going to films, having a television, piercing and tattoos, alcohol and drugs, contraception, and so forth—in other words, avoidance of worldliness and sin (Hoglund 1980, 366; Alanen 1981; Foltz and Yliniemi 2005). Idle hands are regarded a disgrace, if not a sin. Believing that "empty hands do evil things," Anna seldom sat still and never wasted time.

She had to leave school during the fifth grade to help at home. As her siblings got older, Anna began to work outside the home doing domestic work and caring for others' children to bring in money. In her teens, she began to take jobs as a domestic for wealthy and professional families farther from home (Penti 1986; Lindstrom-Best 1988). It wasn't an easy or happy life. Finnish Americans were regarded locally as equivalent to Native Americans, and like Native Americans, these female Finnish workers were often mistreated. At twenty-one, a wiser Anna went to work in Chicago, as did many young Finnish American women. Memories of this time are usually positive: groups of girls from home would rent a room on their day off (usually a Thursday) and have a slumber party. In Chicago, Finnish Americans gained a reputation, I was told, as good, skilled hard workers. They went from one wealthy family to another until they found one that treated them well. Anna had several unpleasant experiences working for families until 1933, when she landed a position as a live-in housekeeper and cook for two sisters who were ophthalmologists. With her earnings, she managed to save her family's farm in the Upper Peninsula. This period is when she began to quilt after seeing quilts on the beds of her employers. Anna loved these women, but after nine happy years, she had to return to the Upper Peninsula because of family illness. However, she returned to these women every Thanksgiving until their deaths in late 1990s; during the holiday, she cooked dinner and polished the silver.

Back home, it was more hard work. She married her longtime sweetheart in 1944, had twin boys, was widowed in 1948, and went to work as a cook in the local school and hospital to support her sons. In 1953, she married a family friend.

Needless to say, during these many years, Anna did not have time to weave. Despite her difficult life, she recalled that all she ever really wanted were "raspberries in my own yard and my own loom." She got both. In 1956 at the age of forty-seven and after thirty-four years away from weaving, she acquired her first loom, a two-harness Union No. 36 that she purchased for $75. (Later, she acquired an Orco, a LeClerc, and a Newcomb.) Her life, however, didn't get easier. Her husband developed Alzheimer's in the 1970s and for twelve years Anna cared for him. Weaving was an important outlet at this time. After his death, Anna had a triple bypass, a procedure she said she'd *never* go through again!

As an Apostolic Lutheran and a child of immigrants who knew poverty, Anna never ever wasted anything. She was frugal, hardworking, and conservative and did not condone or participate in our disposable society. This is what defined Anna. She was the consummate recycler who relished making something out of nothing. As a cook in the school, for example, she baked bread every day for the kids, who tore off the crust and left it on the table. Anna gathered up these leavings, moistened them, and used them in the next day's bread (a sourdough starter). She built her own summer cottage near Lake Superior, but to do so, she needed lumber. Therefore, Anna baked chocolate cake for men at the lumberyard in exchange for boards. She learned millinery from a local hat maker and made hats out of the fur coats and collars she acquired from her employers. For her textile arts, she never used anything other than old fabrics she found in local thrift stores. Her pleasure in making beautiful, useful items from discards began with the hunt. She prowled thrift stores and loved to tell about these adventures, about the treasures she found, and what she was able to make with her findings. She made unique blankets out of coats that she took apart and reconstructed like a jigsaw puzzle, embellishing them with colorful yarn that tied the top to the back that was made from woolen skirt material and multihued bindings around the outer edge. Her handsome braided five- and seven-strand carpets are also made from old coats. And, of course, her woven rag rugs are rich colorful testaments of her ethnicity, ethics, and values.

When Anna finally got her loom, she joined the local weaving and craft guild to brush up on her skills. She very much liked her instructor and learned new weaving techniques. Many of the members of this local guild were local Finns, some very accomplished, some taught at the local college, and all were, of course, familiar with rag rugs. At one meeting, Anna, who was known as a rag rug weaver, was asked by another member if she was still "wasting her time on those old rags." Insulted, Anna quit the guild. She said the fancy weaving she learned there was only good for putting on the wall. She believed in truly functional art works—for instance, rag rugs.

Psychiatrist Gene Cohen (2001) stated that senior creative activity is an impetus for psychological growth and development in the second half of life. The impetus for Anna came a bit later.

The Smithsonian and the Michigan State University Museum were gearing up for the American Folklife Festival when Michigan was to be the featured state in 1987. Anna was selected to represent the Upper Peninsula with Finnish Ameri-

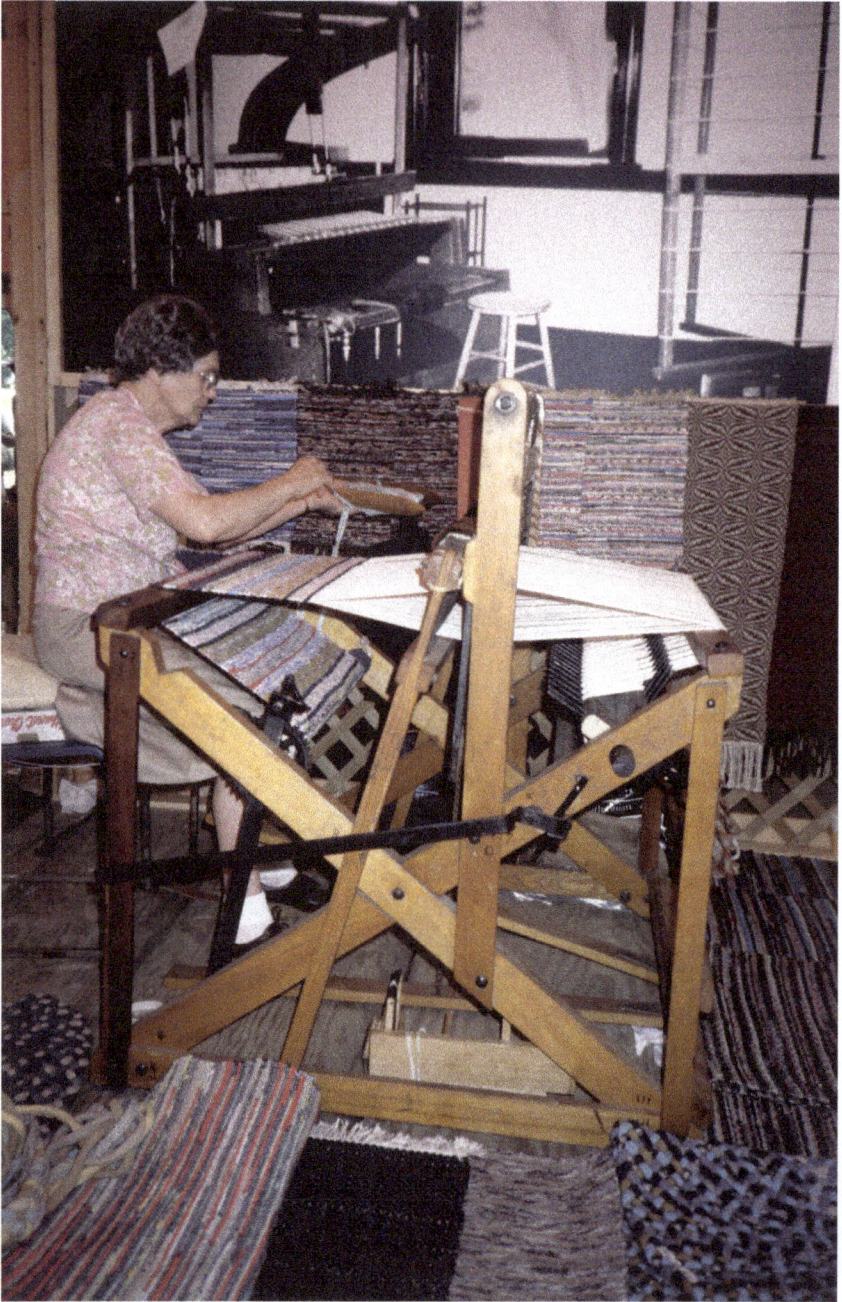

Fig. 5.1. Anna Lassila, at the 1987 American Folklife Festival representing Michigan. *Photograph by Yvonne Lockwood. Courtesy of Michigan State University Museum.*

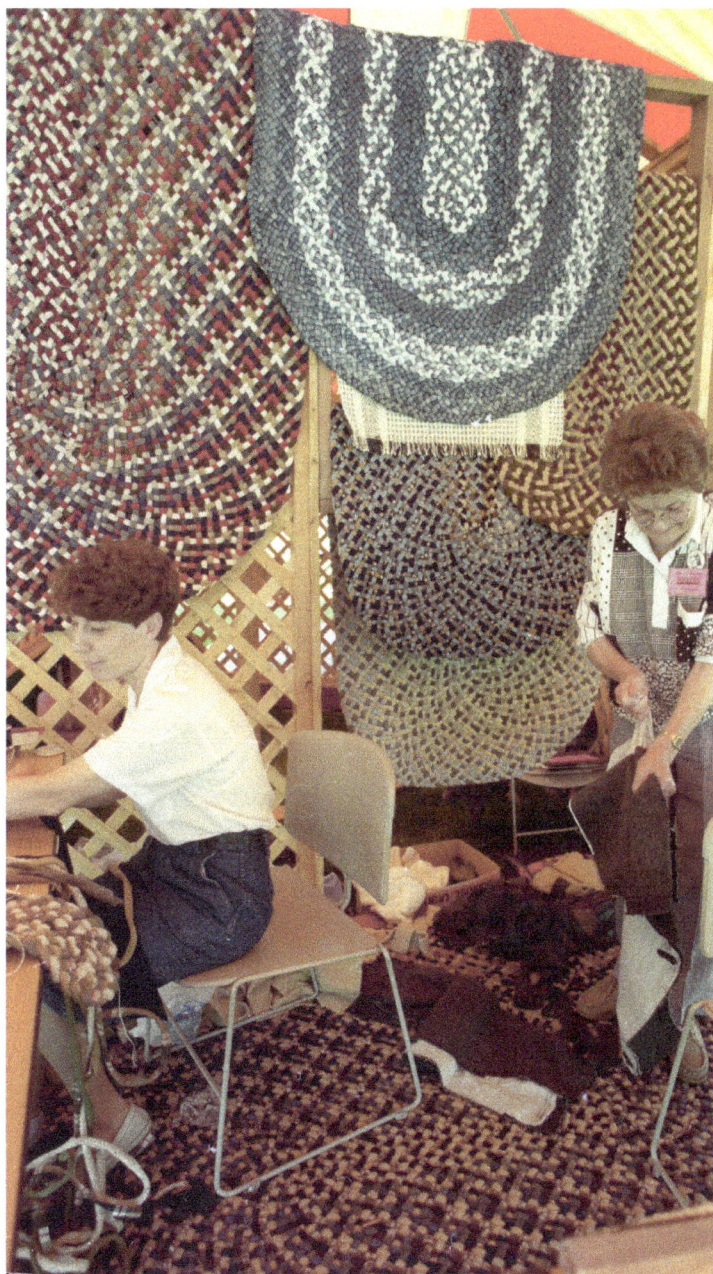

Fig. 5.2. Anna Lassila and Lorri Oikarinen, at the Festival of Michigan Folklife demonstrating multistrand braided rugs. *Photograph by Pearl Wong. Courtesy of Michigan State University Museum.*

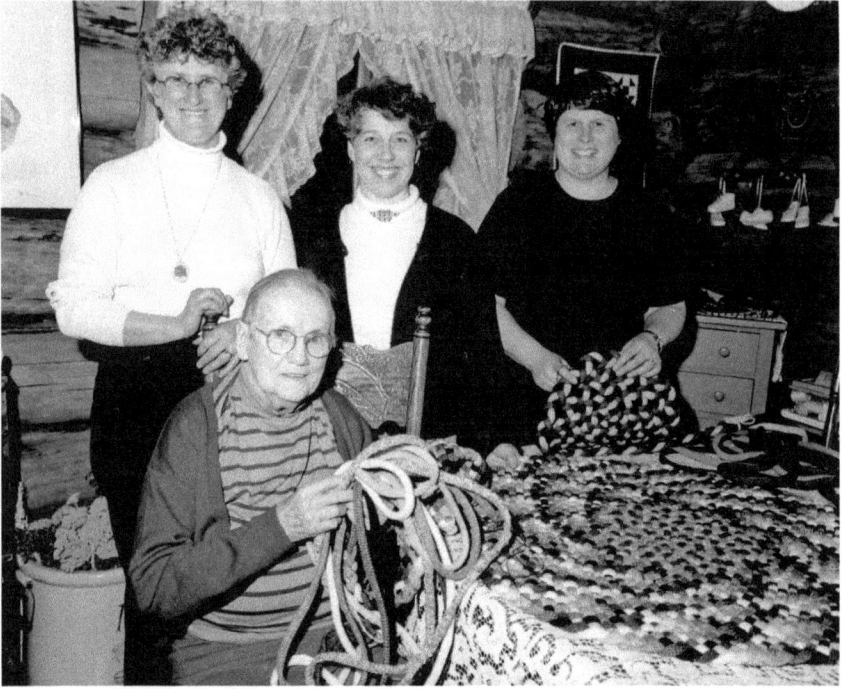

Fig. 5.3. After Anna's stroke, she was unable to teach rug making, but she was included in all the sessions taught by her student, Lorri Oikarinen. (Vivian Huotari, Lorri Oikarinen, Carol Saari, left to right; Anna in front.) *Courtesy of Michigan State University Museum.*

can foods and rag rug weaving. When invited, her response was, "Why me? I'm not good enough." It took a lot of convincing by me and her sons. This energetic, feisty octogenarian was a big hit. The Smithsonian staff spoiled her, the audience adored her, and Anna had the time of her life. Anna returned to the Upper Peninsula overwhelmed. She blossomed with a new self-awareness but never lost her humbleness (fig. 5.1).

Anna had always been appreciated locally; people lined up for her rugs. Although she did occasionally sell her extras, Anna was not a production weaver and she got tired of being pestered to sell. She once told me she was tempted to lie when people asked her if she had rugs to sell. However, appreciation by outsiders has a different impact than that of locals. Her new admirers were folklorists, scholars, and artists—people who regarded her as an artist.

Now Anna began to think about teaching her textile skills to those other than family. She met Lorri Oikarinen of Calumet. Lorri was already an accomplished quilter and weaver with degrees from Michigan State University. They decided to apply for an apprenticeship from the Michigan State University Mu-

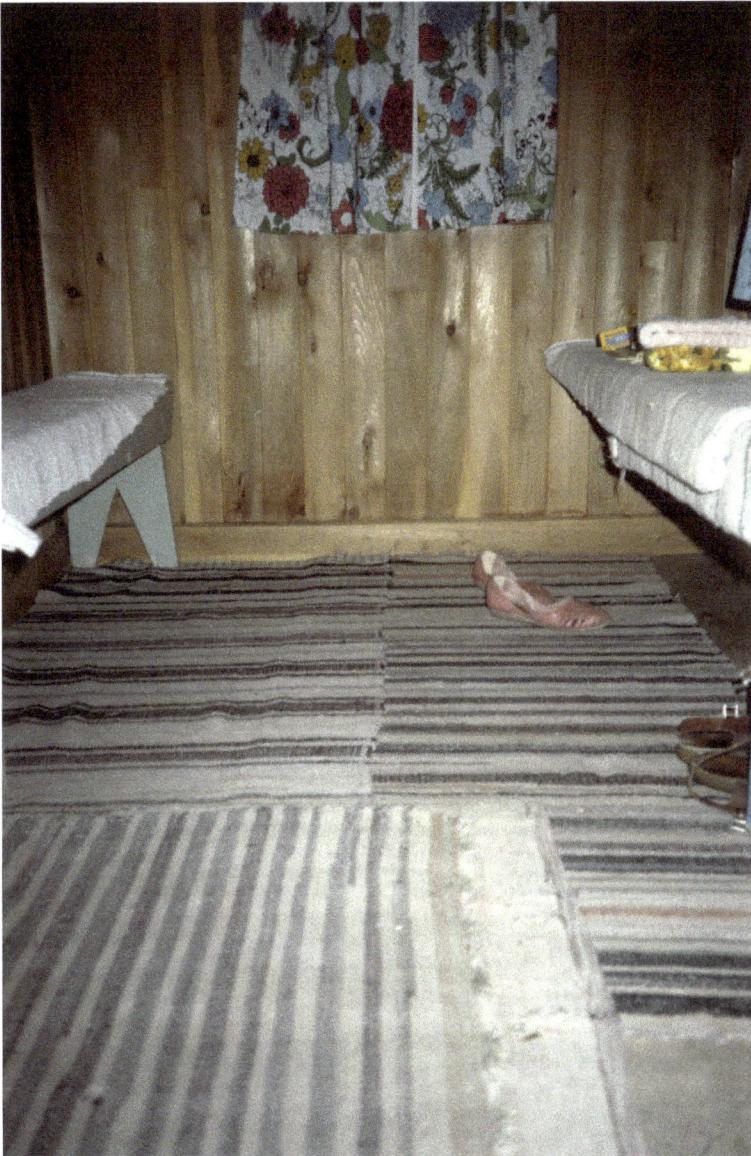

Fig. 5.4. Examples of rag rugs in Anna's sauna dressing room. *Courtesy of Michigan State University Museum.*

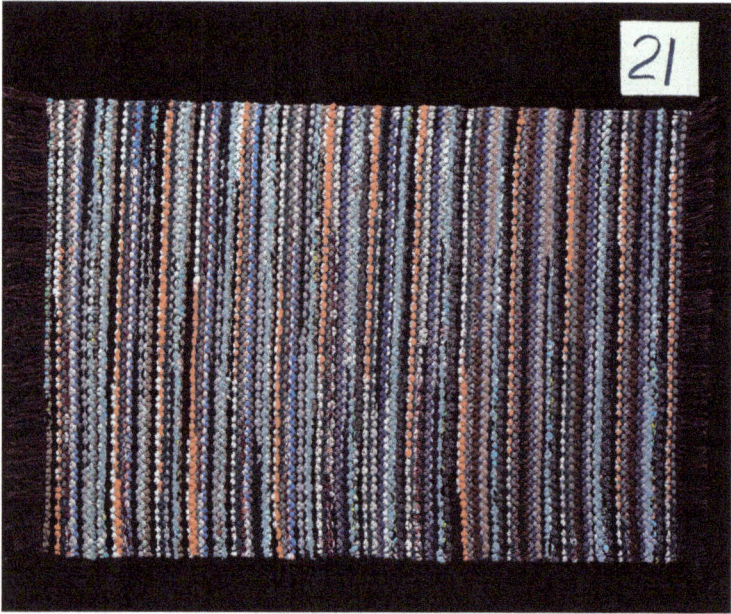

Fig. 5.5. Rag rug. *Courtesy of Michigan State University Museum.*

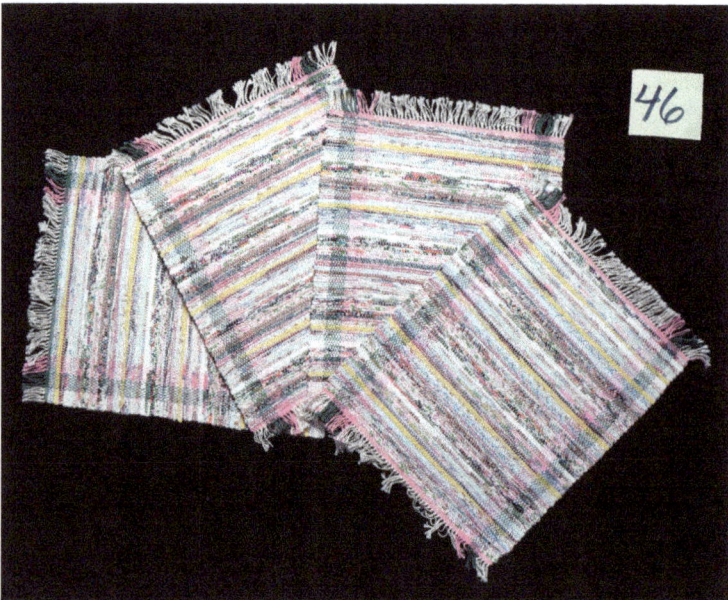

Fig. 5.6. Anna's placemats. *Courtesy of Michigan State University Museum.*

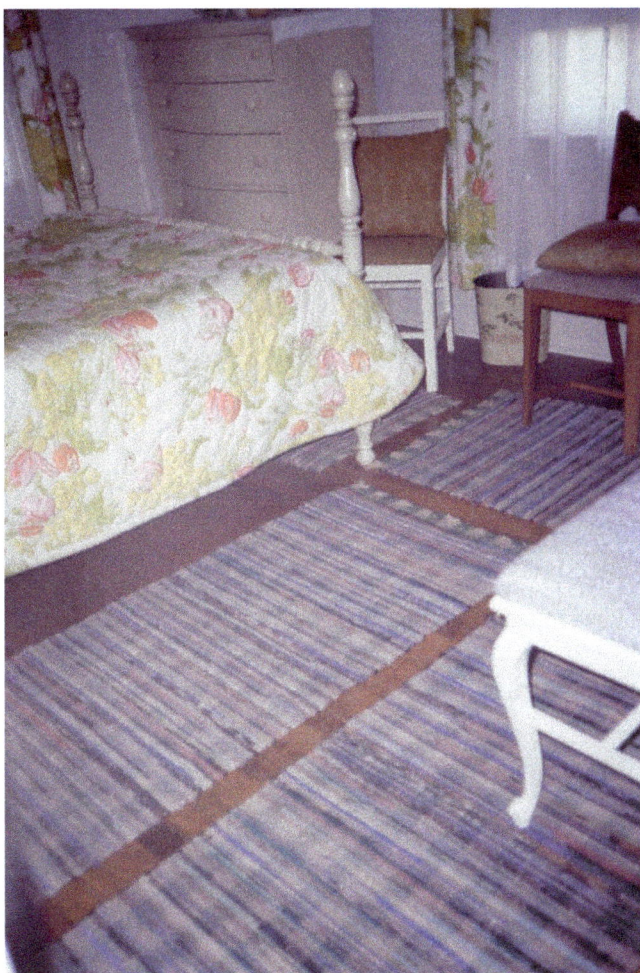

Fig. 5.7. Anna's bedrooms. *Photograph by Yvonne Lockwood. Courtesy of Michigan State University Museum.*

seum's Traditional Arts Program to teach Anna's techniques, values, and aesthetics of rag rug weaving to Lorri. This was the beginning of a very long friendship. Lorri frequently visited Anna; each visit taught her more about Anna and her approach to her art. With a second apprenticeship, Anna taught Lorri her method of five- and seven-strand braided wool rugs. In addition, she held workshops on multistrand braided rugs and demonstrated rug weaving at various events.

Life after the American Folklife Festival was anything but boring. Anna participated with Lorri several times at the Festival of Michigan Folklife (now the

Great Lakes Folk Festival). She was featured in books, newspapers, and magazines (fig. 5.2). Her work was displayed in galleries and museum exhibits. In 1993, she was honored with a Michigan Heritage Award (Kamuda 1996; Lockwood and MacDowell 2004; Lockwood 2010).

Anna had a longtime goal to teach her niece, Vivian, braided and woven rug making. When Vivian moved back to the Upper Peninsula and was ready for instruction, Anna had a debilitating stroke. She was not able to speak and, of course, not able to teach. Because of the apprenticeship program, however, there was someone who could pass on Anna's teachings. Lorri received an apprenticeship award to teach Vivian and another local rag rug weaver braided rugs. They included Anna in all their sessions (fig. 5.3). Although not able to speak, Anna could make herself understood. When students needed correcting Anna let them know by hand gestures and facial expressions.

That was Anna's last time in the creativity arena. In her last year, she lived during the week in a nursing home; her room contained only one of her rag rugs and a few family pictures. But every week Vivian took her to her home for sauna and a familiar environment where she was surrounded by her many creations (fig. 5.4). Her home was like a museum display of her creativity. Looms were set up in the living room and basement. Floors were covered by rag rugs, beds by quilts, windows by lace curtains (figs. 5.5 and 5.6). Walls displayed her "fancy" weaving and crewel work, and her upholstery skills were visible on the furniture (fig. 5.7).[3]

Anna died in 2001. Lorri remembers Anna as a mentor who gave her valuable gifts. A textile artist herself, she stated, "Anna had a heart and soul for her art. Some just slap things together—not Anna. She was a perfectionist and whatever she made had to be pretty. Her rugs are legendary in our area. She had a wonderful sense of color; she used whatever she had and made it work."

Anna Lassila is one of many elders to defy the prevailing negative view of seniors. Her enthusiastic performance of Finnish traditions helped her navigate issues that can beset older adults. Anna said, "I don't have time to be bored." The attention from folklorists and other outsiders to her rugs, coat blankets, quilts, delicious Finnish meals, and other traditions gave Anna a greater sense of her mastery. She wasn't more creative in her eighties, but she had a more acute awareness of her skills and accomplishments and their role in Finnish America.

With her creative work, Anna formed new personal relationships. Through teaching and gifting, she formed bonds of friendship. Anna's art connected her to her Finnish heritage. Her creativity made her Finnish past a meaningful part of her senior years. Her story is about skills that were born of necessity and brought into full bloom in her later years. Anna just got a lot of joy from teaching others, seeing her works on museum walls and galleries, and participating in festivals. She knew she was leaving a legacy.

YVONNE R. LOCKWOOD is Curator Emerita at the Michigan State University Museum. She is author of *Finnish American Rag Rugs: Art, Tradition, Ethnicity.*

## Works Cited

Alanen, Arnold R. 1981. "In Search of the Pioneer Homesteader in America." *Finnish Americana: A Journal of Finnish American History and Culture* 4: 72–92.

Cohen, Gene D. 2001. *The Creative Age: Awakening Human Potential in the Second Half of Life.* New York: Harper Collins.

Foltz, Aila, and Miriam Yliniemi. 2005. *A Godly Heritage: Historical View of the Laestadian Revival and Development of the Apostolic Lutheran Church in America.* Frazee, MN: self-published.

Hoglund, A. William. 1960. *Finnish Immigrants in America, 1880–1920.* Madison: University of Wisconsin Press.

Hoglund, A. William. 1980. "Finns." In *Harvard Encyclopedia of American Ethnic Groups*, edited by Stephen Thernstrom, 366. Cambridge, MA: Harvard University Press.

Hufford, Mary, Marjorie Hunt, and Steve Zeitlin. 1987. *The Grand Generation.* Washington, DC: Smithsonian Institute.

Kamuda, Al. 1996. *Hands across Michigan: Tradition Bearers.* Detroit: Detroit Free Press.

Kay, Jon. 2016. *Folk Art and Aging: Life-Story Objects and Their Makers.* Bloomington: Indiana University Press.

Lindstrom-Best, Varpu. 1988. *Defiant Sisters: A Social History of Finnish Immigrant Women in Canada.* Toronto: Multicultural History Society of Ontario.

Lockwood, Yvonne R. 2010. *Finnish American Rag Rugs: Art, Tradition, and Ethnic Continuity.* East Lansing: Michigan State University Press.

Lockwood, Yvonne, and Marsha MacDowell. 2004. *Honoring Traditions: Michigan Heritage Awards, 1985–2004.* East Lansing: Michigan State University Museum.

Penti, Marsha. 1986. "Piikajutut: Stories Finnish Maids Told." In *Women Who Dared: The History of Finnish American Women*, edited by Carl Ross and Marianne Wargelin Brown, 55–72. St. Paul, MN: Immigration History Research Center.

Schuldiner, David. 1994. "Promoting Self-Worth among the Elderly." In *Putting Folklore to Use*, edited by Michael Owen Jones, 214–25. Lexington: University Press of Kentucky.

## Notes

1. I first met Anna in preparation for the American Folklife Festival in 1986. She came to my attention through the work of Marsha Penti. She seemed to adopt me, and when she spent winters with her son in southeast Michigan and when I went to the Upper Peninsula, we visited. She made certain that I had samples of all her work. When she decided I needed a braided wool rug under my dining room table, she moved in, and for five days and nights we worked to accomplish this task.

2. For a comprehensive study of the Finnish American community in the early years of immigration, see Hoglund (1960).

3. As Jon Kay states, home displays have been ignored by scholars, yet they are prevalent in many ethnic homes, including those of Finnish Americans. These objects are not necessarily made by the homeowners, nor are they always traditional. They are, nonetheless, iconic items, possibly acquired from shops in Finland or Finnish America representing Finnish heritage (Kay 2016, 93).

# 6 Still Working

*Performing Productivity through Gardening and Home Canning*

Danille Elise Christensen

In 2005, Princeton University researchers reported that Americans stereo-type seniors as "warm and incompetent," "dear but doddering"—much like Winnie the Pooh, that silly old bear. In fact, these researchers found that the more inept old people appeared to be—the less independent, intelligent, skillful, or self-confident—the more endearing they seemed to college students, among others. Apparently, younger people in the United States view elders as no threat to their own status, seeing them through a lens of pity rather than with envy, contempt, or admiration (Cuddy, Norton, and Fiske 2005).[1]

This condescension toward elders is increasingly common. Medical progress and other demographic factors have led to large senior cohorts; in response, mandatory retirement ages have been imposed in many parts of the world, effectively institutionalizing obsolescence. Today, elders are also less relevant to the acquisition of knowledge, as population mobility takes young people out of the daily orbit of their grandparents and instructional media shift the ways that hands-on learning happens. In addition, "accelerated technological innovation" encourages continual procurement of new material goods, skills, and knowledge, rather than the application of familiar lived experience (Esposito 1987, 121; Myer-hoff 1992; Cuddy, Norton, and Fiske 2005).[2]

Home food production and preservation is one area of cultural practice that illustrates these trends, their consequences, and their future implications. Historically, small-scale foodwork has been a way for seniors to remain physically, economically, creatively, and socially active, especially in rural areas where social

*The Expressive Lives of Elders* (2018): 106–137, DOI: 10.2979/expressivelivesofelders.0.0.07

structures have encouraged "complementarity and mutual dependence between the generations" (Halperin 1990, 45). In northeastern Kentucky, for instance, anthropologist Rhoda Halperin (1990, 45) has observed that "elderly people perform important management, production, and food-processing tasks," especially with regard to gardening and canning; in many parts of the United States, these activities enact cultural priorities, including "a widely held value placed on self-sufficiency and independence" (Quandt 1994, 198).

However, women in particular have had to contend with negative public perceptions of "the grandmother" and with expert discourses that actively construe women's traditional knowledge as skill-less or even dangerous. Drawing on archived interviews and public discourse, this essay explores the motivations for pursuing food production after age fifty-five, suggests how these activities get mislabeled or disrupted, and highlights some interventions meant to encourage traditional forms of food production and distribution.[3]

## "That's the Main Thing: Work"

In their book *Successful Aging*, John Rowe and Robert Kahn (1998, 169) define productive behavior as "any activity, paid or unpaid, that generates goods or services of economic value"—including tasks completed at home and in the community, such as making meals or keeping an eye on one's neighbor. Yet, the often gendered labor of everyday carework does not command a wage or social respect on par with other kinds of productive labor (Brownlee 1979; DeVault 1991; Meyer 2000; Sayer, Freedman, and Bianchi 2016; Vanek 1979), and indeed these activities are sometimes entirely excluded from the category "work."[4] Variables such as age also affect the ways people conceptualize valuable work: even as many Americans assume that the old should relinquish their jobs to the young, we also imagine unemployed seniors as a burden, a population rooted in dependency (Antonucci et al., 2016, 52; Esposito 1987, 218–19; Morrow-Howell and Greenfield 2016; Rowe and Kahn 1998, 168).

Still, many elders want to be up and doing, and they count work as a core value and obligation. Hershel Clay Hatton (b. 1936) of Estill County, Kentucky, said this about his college-bound grandchildren: "It tickles me. I don't care what they do just as long as they work. That's the main thing: work" (Hatton 2012, 9). He himself began paid employment as a teenager, first farming with horses, then taking jobs in a sawmill, as an electrician, in the oil fields, as a truck driver. And for more than fifty years, he and his wife, Wanda, had also kept a garden. "Hard work won't kill you," Hatton said, and he should know. "Still out here gardening," mused the seventy-five-year-old in a 2012 interview (Hatton 2012, 11).

Arlene Flynn Chaney (b. 1933), four years Hatton's senior, was also born and raised in Estill County; she started gardening as a child. Later, as an adult fully

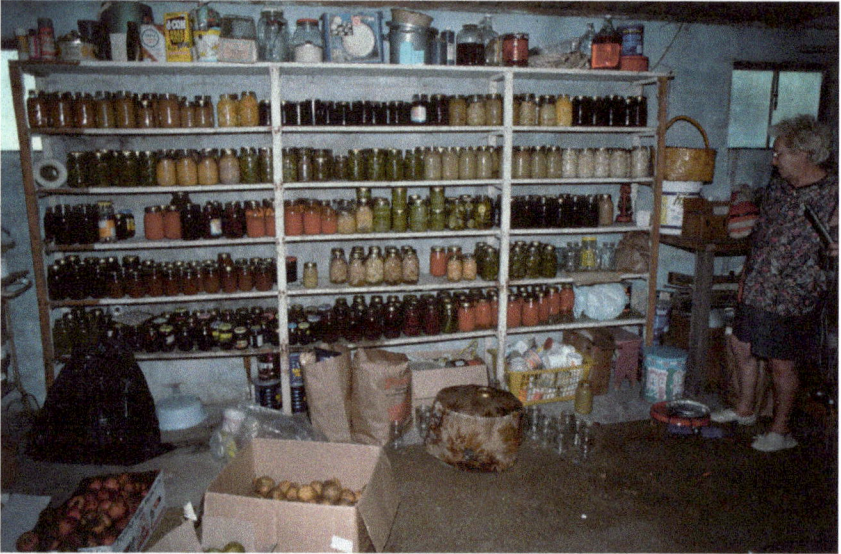

Fig. 6.1. *Sadie Miller with Produce from Gardens and Woods Preserved in Her Basement Pantry. Photograph by Lyntha Scott Eiler, Drews Creek, West Virginia, September 1995. Coal River Folklife Collection (AFC 1999/008), American Folklife Center, Library of Congress, Washington, DC. CRF-LE-C017-11.*

aware of her own skills and preferences, she chose not to "fool with" some kinds of labor, such as making candy or chocolate gravy. And she'd abandoned red-eye gravy—conjured from coffee and pork drippings—per doctors' orders. By 2012, when she was interviewed for an Appalachian foodways project, her diabetic husband had lost his hearing and was losing his eyesight; she also endured limited mobility, because she rarely drove. But gardening was a different matter: "I just like to be out there, you know," she said. Activity kept her mind and spirit healthy. "I guess it's year before last I thought I wouldn't put out a garden, and seem like I just got so depressed and I was wanting, you know, something to do besides [being] in the house all the time." Laughing, she reported, "And finally I said, 'Well, we need us a little garden plowed up'" (Chaney 2012, 33). Hard work was not an issue: Chaney liked growing labor-intensive strawberries the best, especially because they were one of the few foods her young granddaughter would eat.[5] She also wanted to keep busy: "I find they's something you gotta do in the garden every day" (Chaney 2012, 36).

Processing these garden goods can be a daily occupation, too. In 1995, Sadie Ellis Cool Miller (b. 1916) of Drews Creek, West Virginia, told folklorist Mary Hufford that she served something she'd canned or frozen herself at the table nearly every day (fig. 6.1). Producing and preserving food—even if she already had plenty stored away—was "something I was raised to do," she said; her mother had set her to picking blackberries as a small child in Clifftop, West Virginia. In fact, she remarked with a smile, her husband Howard had refused to plant anything but tomatoes the summer before she was interviewed. He had explained, "If I'da planted a garden, you'da worked yourself to death trying to put it all up" (S. Miller 1995).

To be known as a hard worker is a high compliment in many parts of the United States. During her fieldwork in the Allegheny foothills of West Virginia, for instance, Katherine Roberts explored how the products of work—garden produce, dressed meat, home-bottled goods—demonstrated both aesthetic and ethical competence. These processes and objects stand as evidence of versatility and inventiveness, a way to demonstrate specialized knowledge and personal foresight, and the means for contributing to networks of reciprocity (Roberts 2006; Halperin 1990). In other words, producing and preserving food can be an important way to maintain and display continuing relevance, even in old age.[6]

## "I Can Survive When the Electric's Out"

Home food production is a cultural and a social practice particularly in rural areas, where it has long been part of a "system of local knowledge and practices that allows people to exercise control over their livelihood" and experience other kinds of autonomy (Halperin 1990, 11). One survey conducted in rural Kentucky among people fifty-five and older found that 56 percent of 639 respondents raised home gardens during summer 1990, with little difference in gardening activity between those in mountainous and flat terrain. Of those gardeners, 84 percent also canned at least some of their produce, and 80 percent froze some of it. A quarter of the overall sample also bought or were gifted at least one item of garden produce—especially green beans and tomatoes—and the nongardeners were likely to preserve these food gifts (Quandt 1994).

Elders who grow and preserve food are often building on their own previous experience. In-depth interviews with twenty participants in the 1990 study revealed "large and diverse" gardens from childhood, even in coal camps (Quandt 1994, 195). A decade later, a study of 145 community-dwelling seniors in rural central North Carolina found that its equal numbers of white, black, and indigenous participants regularly recounted family norms of self-sufficiency, naming food production and management techniques as essential for dealing with circumstances that included large families, small salaries, and economic and natural disasters (Quandt et al. 2001). A more recent study in rural southwest Virginia, though modest in scope, is consistent with findings in other rural communities. All fourteen people—mostly seniors—interviewed in 2015 as part of a

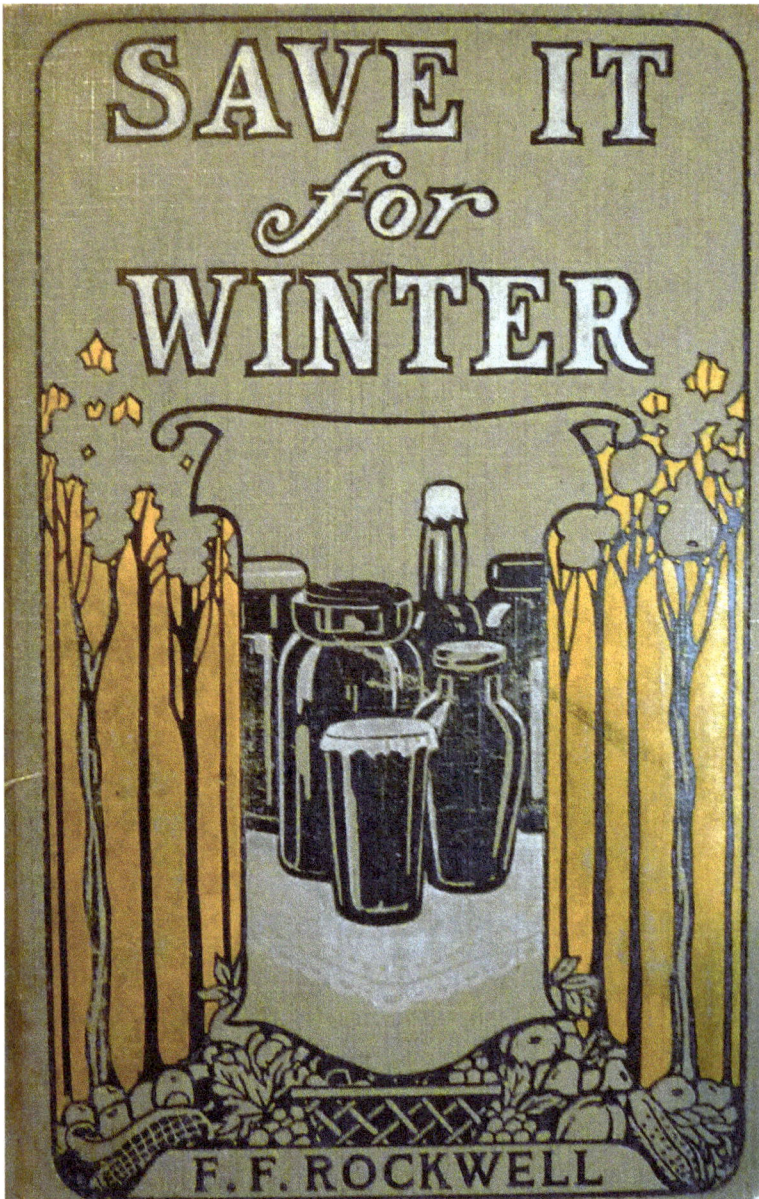

Fig. 6.2. Frederick Frye Rockwell's *Save It for Winter: Modern Methods of Canning, Dehydrating, Preserving and Storing Vegetables and Fruit for Winter Use, with Comments on the Best Things to Grow for Saving, and When and How to Grow Them* (New York: Frederick A. Stokes Company, 1918) extolled home bottling as an efficient, economical, healthy, and moral response to conditions attending the Great War.

container gardening program in Grayson County, Virginia, linked themselves in a meaningful way to "a past agricultural narrative" that included gardening and food preservation (fig. 6.2). Further, most were still embedded in family and community home food production networks (Dobson 2016, 14).[7] Recalling her natal family's norms, sixty-three-year-old Ada remembered, "Even if you lost your job, you could still eat. Those cans and that garden, you won't go hungry." Terri, age seventy, recalled, "We picked a lot . . . by hand, did a lot of canning. . . . I can survive when the electric's out." Skills related to food production, combined with knowledge of and access to alternative technologies such as oil lamps, wood stoves, and water wells, gave participants confidence in their own ability to be independent (Dobson 2016, 77).

Historically, home food production has also facilitated economic self-sufficiency: market stands or informal exchanges generate cash income and bolster family budgets (e.g., Halperin 1990). In 2015, older residents in southwest Virginia noted that homegrown vegetables were at least half as expensive as store-bought ones and often of better quality—important considerations during a time when everyone was "having a hard time making ends meet" (Dobson 2016, 84).

## "I Dearly Love to Do It"

Although economic imperatives favor maintaining kitchen or subsistence gardens, "craft satisfaction"—pride in a materially productive task well done—is also an important motivation (Strasser 1982). Reputations may be established as people dig in the dirt. In northeastern Kentucky, retired milk inspector Alfred Jones and his wife turned to truck[8] farming, selling homegrown corn, tomatoes, zucchini, cabbage, broccoli, eggplant, and okra at their summer market stand in order to buy groceries for themselves. But the enterprise was also a chance to display skill (fig. 6.3): Jones developed "a regular regional clientele who [knew] him for his prizes at the county fair" (Halperin 1990, 83; cf. Marsden 2010 and Prosterman 1995).

Aesthetic pleasure also contributes to quality of life, both physically and psychologically. Increasingly, researchers in the field of geriatrics are focusing on skills, strengths, and satisfactions of older adults, rather than dwelling on signs and symptoms of degeneration. They have found positive health impacts of creative expression, including the benefits of a sense of mastery—which improves immune system function—and sustained social relationships—which reduce stress markers, depression, and medication use, and increase brain resilience (Cohen 2006).

Of course, food gardening also has an impact on nutrition. For instance, some seniors prefer the taste of homegrown foods despite the time and effort involved in creating them. Rita Rae Higgins (b. 1937) lived much of her childhood in West Virginia's panhandle, where her mother worked in a steel plant, but spent

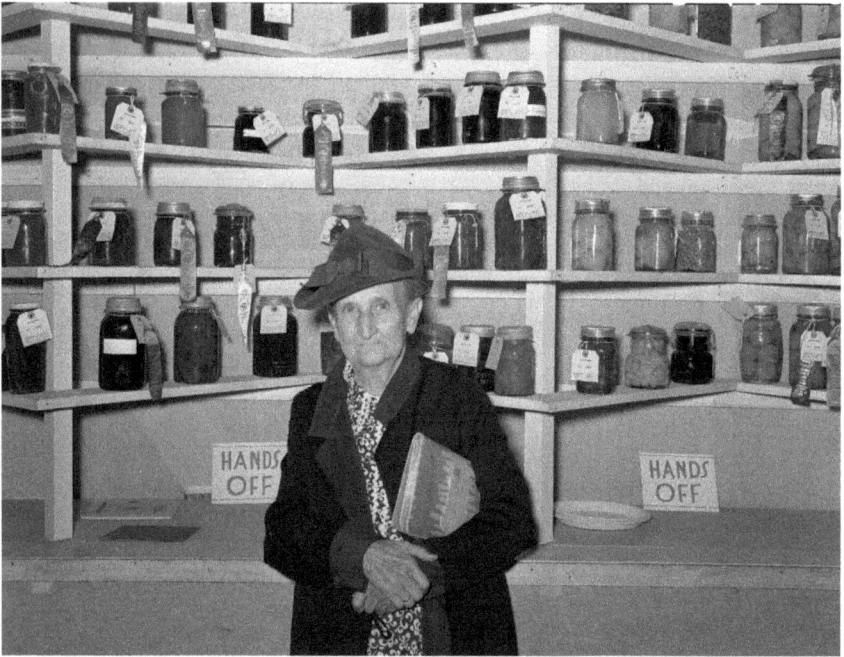

Fig. 6.3. Aesthetic pleasure—taste, smell, color—can be another motivation for productivity, as evidenced by careful public displays like this one at the Gonzales County Fair. *Photograph by Russell Lee, Gonzales, Texas, 1939. FSA/OWI Collection, Prints and Photographs Division, Library of Congress, Washington, DC. LC-USF34-034584-D.*

summers with her grandparents in Pleasants County, West Virginia, where she had been born. Both grandmothers put her to work washing jars and peeling fruit, and Higgins's mother used her vacation time to can with her parents on the farm, then take half the finished jars home to Weirton. As an adult, Higgins moved back to Pleasants County to work in a care facility for people with mental disabilities. Interviewed in 2012 at age seventy-four, she was growing tomatoes in pots and cucumbers in a child's sandbox. It had become too difficult to till her own ground, but she was still canning, buying bulk produce at the farmers' markets and managing to squeeze one batch of pickles out of the sandbox cukes: "We do like the home-canned pickles the best," she said (Higgins 2012, 7). Other seniors who gardened, even in this limited way, reported that the practice impacted their diet: better tasting, readily available produce meant that they consumed more fresh food during the growing season (Dobson 2016, 76).

Some find the predictable work of gardening and food preparation soothing. In Grayson County, Virginia, fifty-five-year-old Gloria said, "I like the feel of dirt between my toes. . . . It's very therapeutic to have it in your hands." Terri con-

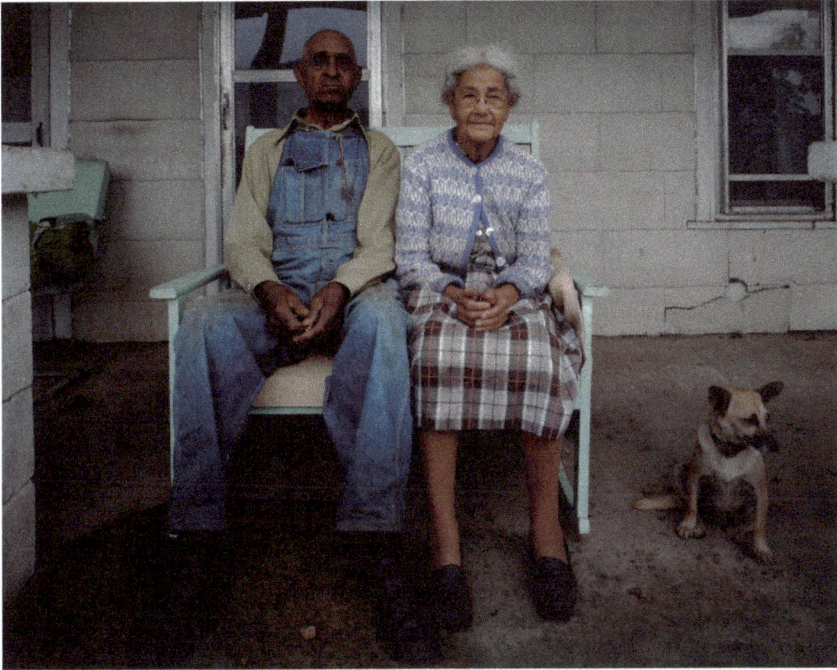

Fig. 6.4. In 1978, Pat Mullen interviewed Mamie and Leonard Bryan on their farm near Sparta, North Carolina, which had been bought with money Leonard earned in West Virginia coal mines. Mamie tended the children and the farm in his absence. When Mullen visited, he found shelves and a chest freezer full of preserved fruit, vegetables, and meat. *Portrait of Mamie and Leonard Bryan. Photograph by Terry Eiler. Blue Ridge Parkway Folklife Project Collection (AFC 1982/009), American Folklife Center, Library of Congress, Washington, DC. BR-8-TE-151/4.*

curred: "The peace and the quiet, just by yourself working in it, thinking, talking to God, playing in the dirt . . . it's just calming. It helps you" (Dobson 2016, 76). Sadie Miller, in West Virginia's Coal River Valley, said that bottling produce became more fun than work, given adequate knowledge and skill. The hardest part about canning beets was harvesting them, she said—and her neighbor Roy Webb had already completed that labor for her. After boiling the beets, "well, it's a lotta fun to stand there and peel 'em like that, you know": the skins slipped right off when rubbed. She enjoyed the tidy displays made possible by such a bright mess. "I dearly love to do it," Miller said. "I like in the wintertime to see all that good stuff" (S. Miller 1995).

Finally, the pleasure of witnessing accumulation, of "watching things grow," was voiced by many participants in the 2015 container gardening interviews. Forty-three-year-old Carl echoed some of the older study participants who appreciated producing something measurable: "I get a thrill out of how big [plants] can get, you know, how much you can get off them" (Dobson 2016, 76). Arlene Chaney also cultivated quantity. Her mother always had preserves ready for the family's hot breakfast biscuits, and Chaney developed a "weakness" for jams and jellies. As her fruits and berries came on, she'd "put up a little at a time." But in 2012 she had resolved not to buy any more canning jars because she'd run out of room: "First thing you know you got a terrible lot put up, and then I think it was last year I thought, 'Well, what has become of my pint jars?'" Laughing, she recalled discovering them stacked on her shelves, all already full (Chaney 2012, 18).

## "Share, Share Alike"

These tasty surpluses facilitate traditional community responses to food insecurity and social isolation: food gifting creates and sustains interpersonal resource networks. One 2001 study designed to be generalizable to the southeastern United States found that food gifts—from children, neighbors, and church members—permeated discussions held with seniors in central North Carolina. These gifts, which included fresh and preserved produce, "were considered socially acceptable [forms of assistance] and symbols of community," perhaps because they could be explained as forms of serial reciprocity in a system that seniors had paid into when they themselves were younger (Quandt et al. 2001, 367, 370). Every participant in Liza Dobson's case study in Grayson County, Virginia, said that reciprocal gifting of produce, labor, and tools was a fundamental part of local food cultures. Henry, age seventy-five, remarked, "That's about the way it is around here. And our neighbors, if they don't have something, we give it to them, you know. Share, share alike. . . . That's the way it's supposed to be" (Dobson 2016, 80–81; cf. Christensen 2015 and Puckett 2000).[9]

Thrift and cooperative provisioning link hand in glove here. Carrie Severt, in North Carolina's Blue Ridge Mountains, laughed at the thought of eating through her pantry herself—with her family grown, it would take her and her husband a hundred years, she said, to consume all she'd canned. But she didn't want to waste what other people might need (Severt 1978). Sadie Miller canned green tomatoes and dried squash in part because she also hated to see these items go to waste. Her pantry was a mix of stored and preserved food from neighbors and friends, and she'd had such a big crop of apples in 1995—limbs on the Red Delicious had been in danger of breaking—that after she'd dried some, frozen some, cellared some, and turned others into apple butter, she called for her neighbors to take the rest (S. Miller 1995).

Small-scale food production in the rural lowland and upland South resonates with other sites in which these practices are integrated into dense, multi-

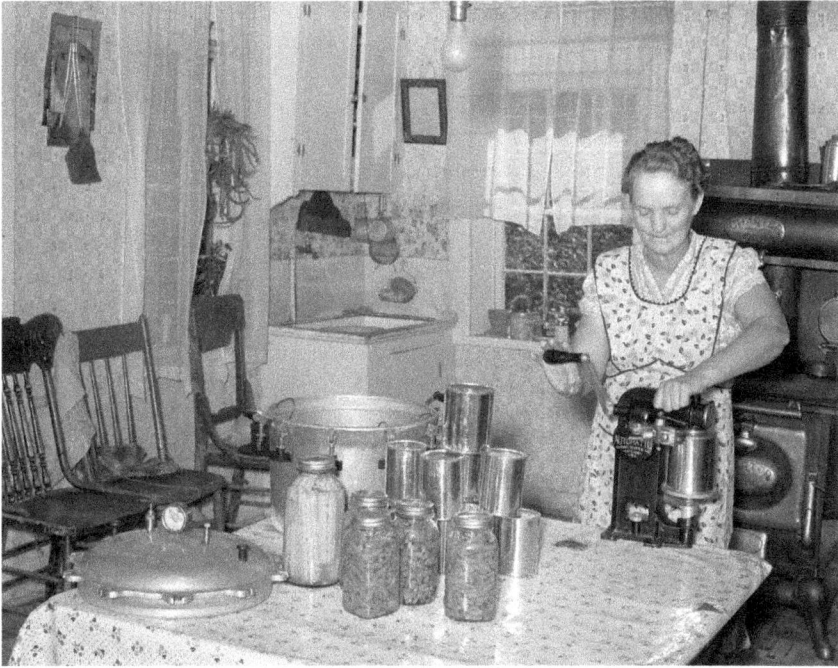

Fig. 6.5. *Mrs. Christiansen of the Christiansen Canning Unit Sealing Cans. During 1939, she canned 2,300 quarts that included twenty mutton, two deer, two beefs, five pigs. Fish was tried very successfully. In this cooperative agreement, there were twenty-five users, and outside of the cooperative, there were ten others who used Mrs. Christiansen's services. Photograph by Russell Lee, Box Elder County, Utah, 1940. FSA/OWI Collection, Prints and Photographs Division, Library of Congress, Washington, DC. LC-USF34-037615-D.*

plex social networks (fig. 6.5).[10] For example, letters written by Lillie Liston Baker (b. 1884) reveal how food preservation organized both her attention and her social life in midcentury Utah. Her archived correspondence with daughter Ruth Thompson, who lived on a cherry orchard and mink farm a few hours north, begins in 1950, when Baker was sixty-six years old. After her husband's death, she had reluctantly moved from her ranch in Boulder to Escalante, a town in southern Utah's red rock district. Unable to drive, she wanted to be surrounded by friends and family, who literally lived next door, across the back fence, and two doors down (Baker 1950–1960).

September letters during the next decade detail the ways Baker and her neighbors pooled resources, ordering from or traveling to fruit-rich areas together in order to obtain produce they couldn't get locally. One year, family members brought eighty quarts of peaches from trees in the area where she'd raised her children; another year, daughter Ruth arranged to send a shipment of peaches and prunes south from her home in Santaquin, the fruit destined to be sugared and bottled by her mother. Family and friends also helped Baker manage the excesses from her own garden. When a son visited from California, she sent him back west with a carload of bottled fruit, vegetables, and frozen beef and venison, and she gifted extra produce to family members and neighbors. On September 13, 1950, Baker reported that her daughter Vonda Pollock had been picking bushels of tomatoes and bottling peaches; Vonda had secured one bushel of grapes for her mother to make into jelly, and Baker reciprocated by giving extra sweet corn to her and to several daughters-in-law. In bumper years like 1954, Baker sent Boulder peaches up to Ruth, along with other goods, including a piano and family documents. Despite having moved off the ranch, Baker was proud of her provisioning. In October 1950, she wrote, "I have all the garden gathered in, have got the pig killed and in the freezer. . . . We got a nice lot of vegetables and fruit bottled most all the bottles are full, plenty in that cellar for two years." When seventy-six-year-old Lillie Baker died in 1960 after a protracted battle with cancer, there was still bottled fruit on her shelves and tomatoes to be picked in the garden (Baker 1950–1960).

Food-based reciprocity involves exchanges of labor as well as goods, as demonstrated by Mary Josephine (Josie) Wilson Bateman's turn-of-the-century diary. Bateman was born in Midway, Utah, in 1877, to an Irish father and a Swiss mother. Her third diary begins in August 1902, just as the early apples were coming on, and it offers an abbreviated account of life with two toddlers and a husband regularly away herding sheep or doing seasonal work such as hoeing sugar beets. Throughout the journals, she uses the terms *putting up* and *bottling*, but also sometimes just calls it *work*. This is work done at the homes of others, often *for* others. In her records, relatives and friends trade food-related labor—such as drying corn or bottling pears—alongside the work of childcare, tending the sick, and organizing celebrations and funerals. Sometimes these co-laborers are her age peers, but often it is parents, aunts and uncles, and older cousins who offer physical assistance as well as a range of fruits from their own orchards and gardens (Bateman 1902–1905).

Similarly, in Brick County, Kentucky, the family of Hattie Kimball (b. 1926) regularly assisted nearby relatives with their tobacco harvests in exchange for aid with domestic labor, including canning. Like Lillie Baker's children, Kimball's also helped her obtain fresh produce (Halperin 1990, 63–64). Mamie Lee Bryan (b. 1898) put up canned and frozen food on the farm near Sparta, North Carolina, that was purchased with money Leonard Bryan (b. ca.1888) earned as he worked in West Virginia coal mines (see fig. 6.4). In her husband's absence, Mamie tended the children, the farm, her flowers, and his mother and brothers; when he was home, Leonard farmed but also plowed gardens for neighbors throughout

Alleghany County. Their children remember him singing "almost to town" as he headed out before dawn to get this work done (Bryan and Bryan 1978; McMillan, Valentine, and Myers 2006).

Such efforts are cyclical and self-replicating. Trading labor and goods helps to establish and maintain social networks, which in turn augment material outputs. Researchers have found that "older adults with more personal and social resources are more likely to be productively engaged" (Morrow-Howell and Greenfield 2016, 302). Further, social connections like these are crucial to individual longevity. Wrote one researcher, "A subjective sense of social isolation predicts mortality as well as smoking a pack of cigarettes a day predicts mortality" (Antonucci et al. 2016, 44; cf. Sayer, Freedman, and Bianchi 2016, 173).

## "She's Learned a Lot from Us, I Think"

One final form of productivity is knowledge transfer: teaching rising generations. Clay Hatton (b. 1936), who plants according to moon phases and other astrological signs, considered this attention to environmental contexts a kind of insurance necessary for those who were "dependent on the Lord for what they had" (2012, 5–6); he himself was the youngest of ten children in a family that felt the effects of the Great Depression into the 1940s and didn't have access to electricity until 1949. In 2012, Hatton continued to grow staples such as cabbage, onions, potatoes, and corn and stocked his pantry with bottled green beans, tomatoes, and pickles. Passing on this knowledge was important to him (cf. Dobson 2016, 80–81). Researchers report that intergenerational knowledge transfer is good for seniors, but in his interview with a Berea College student, Hatton focused mostly on the altruistic aspects of teaching.[11] Referring to a young neighbor, he reflected, "She's learned a lot from us, I think [laughter]. She's canning and doin stuff on her own, and if she don't know something she don't care to askt [i.e., she doesn't mind asking]. . . . She's a workin little ol girl I'll say that for her [laughter]." With three children to raise, he said, "she might need everything that she learns, she'll need every bit of it growin, comin up through life" (Hatton 2012, 7).

The value of this kind of traditional knowledge has sometimes been lauded in broader public talk. Frederick Rockwell, a gardening enthusiast who wrote the 1918 home food preservation manual *Save It for Winter*, suggested that women had learned through experience what scientists had only recently identified: "For generations housewives have known that corn was very hard to keep even if carefully canned. Corn and tomatoes put up together, however, keep very well." The reason, scientists had discovered, was that acid supplied by the tomatoes "makes living conditions which the bacteria refuse to tolerate" (Rockwell 1918, 10; see fig. 6.2). Decades later, a sugar company in the intermountain west validated skills transmitted in practice: a midcentury advertisement in a Mormon women's magazine depicted a young woman preparing award-winning jellies by applying some of her "grandma's know-how." "To get clear shimmering jellies that sparkle in the glass," the ad copy advised, "you've got to combine . . . wholesome, ripe fruit with pure fine granulated sugar . . . possibly some fruit pectin, and a little of grandma's know-how" (Utah-Idaho Sugar 1950).

## "She Might Poison Her Entire Family"

Yet more often, twentieth-century popular discourse has portrayed older women's expertise as either already outdated or on the verge of irrelevance. Even as the Utah-Idaho Sugar Company called on consumers to employ "grandma's know-how," for instance, one midcentury commercial booklet characterized traditional jelly making as "guesswork" conveniently eliminated by the magic of artificial pectin (Certo ca. 1951). Discounted here was all the accumulated knowledge that enabled respected cooks to discern which combination of specific fruits, degree of ripeness, and length and style of cooking would yield a respectably firm preserve. Further, and despite the fact that many actual grandmothers in the last decades of the century defined themselves as youthful, fun-loving, and urbanized, advertisements depicted them as white-haired, bespectacled, and aproned, surrounded by rocking chairs, old-fashioned appliances, and adoring offspring. Consistent with broader norms of condescension toward seniors, twentieth-century ads projected a sense of safety but simultaneously nurtured a suspicion that these protected spaces and practiced skills were out of step with modernity (Johnson 1983; Parkin 2006; fig. 6.6).

Some of these elderly domestic imaginaries were deemed not only dear and doddering but also dangerous. Although home canning can be presented as a feel-good nostalgic practice, industry- and university-based communication about this kind of food preservation has regularly invoked fear of social failure or even physical death. To be sure, people have died from eating hermetically sealed foods stored at room temperature—botulism is a real threat, the result of a toxin produced by a common spore under specific and complexly intertwined conditions. One important variable, for instance, is acid. Most fruits contain enough natural acid to inhibit the *Clostridium botulinum* spore even in the warm, anaerobic conditions in which it thrives—but figs and many new varieties of tomatoes need the assistance of additional acid (e.g., lemon juice) in order to be stored safely in bottled form on the shelf. Unpickled meats and vegetables are so low-acid that they need to be cooked at higher-than-natural boiling points (i.e., above 212° F, in a pressure canner) for specific durations in order to inactivate *C. botulinum* spores.[12] These realizations came about gradually, however, and they happened in conjunction with shifts in what people attempted to can, the equipment they were using to do it, and the ways they used the food after it had been bottled.

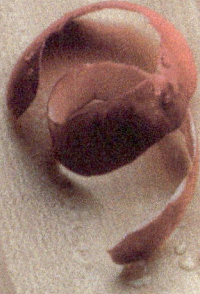

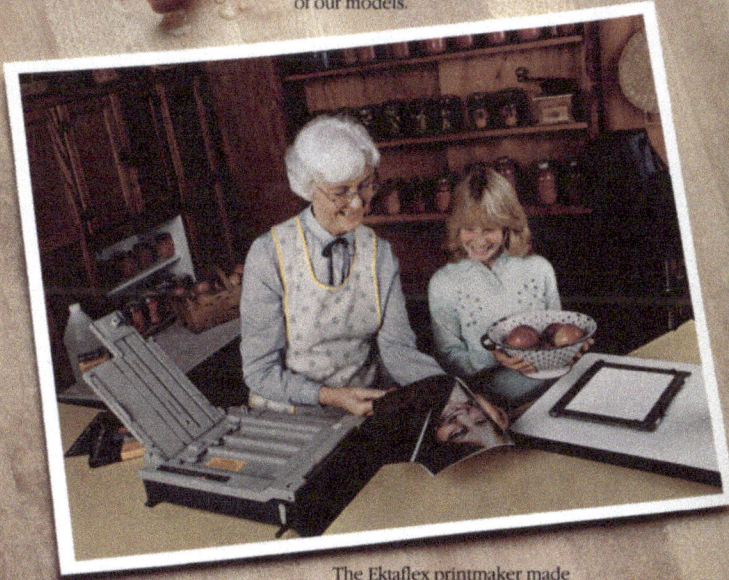

Fig. 6.6. This 1982 advertisement bucks trends by incorporating "modern" equipment but does so by minimizing the complexity of traditional skills. It promotes the Kodak Ektaflex personal printmaker by implying its similarities to the simple processing that occurs in the kitchen: like making a pie or bottling the tomatoes that line the walls of this pantry, the only things would-be developers have to worry about are time and temperature. Even an old lady can do it. Eastman Kodak Co., c. 1982. "As Easy as Apple Pie." *Wolfman Report on the Photographic Industry in the United States, 1981–82*, back cover. New York: Modern Photography Magazine/ABC Leisure Magazines.

The National Center for Home Food Preservation (http://nchfp.uga.edu/) at the University of Georgia regularly publishes important updated recommendations that address these kinds of changes.

Unfortunately, most published discourse does not distinguish contexts of production and use from the identities of food producers; instead, the authority of science is often simply pitted against the ostensible ignorance or inattention of "the housewife." Dangerous methods are tagged as such by linking them to women's knowledge and practice, which is characterized as unthinking repetition and personified in "the grandmother." For instance, the 2007 textbook *Food Safety: Old Habits, New Perspectives* begins a chapter called "Old Habits Die Hard" by recounting (alongside three other told-as-true case studies) a widely circulated legend/rumor/joke about the women in a family cutting off the ends of a roast before cooking it, simply because "Grandma always does it that way." It turns out that a great-grandmother had had to trim the meat in order to fit it into her roasting pan, and her posterity adopted the method as a fundamental truth. In the textbook's retelling—and in similar accounts on leadership and organizational behavior websites—"Grandma" stands in for rote tradition and is cast as a threat to health or to innovation more generally (Entis 2007, 1; cf. Blum 2010; Guest n.d.; Kibbe 2014; Kinnear 2010).[13]

Decades before, in 1935, bacteriologist Fred Tanner had decried homemakers in thrall to advisers who passed on, in his words, "erroneous" information and "faulty" processes. He wrote that while "the art of food preservation in the factory" had never been "on a sounder basis"—no outbreaks of botulism had been linked to American industrially canned goods for ten years—food preserved by American wives, mothers, and grandmothers was not only likely to spoil but also might "poison her entire family" (Tanner 1935, 301, 303). "Those who interpret scientific data for those who are less informed," he implored, "must leave nothing unsaid. Improperly processed home-canned foods are hazardous" (305). Tanner was correct that printed instructions in the first part of the century were inconsistent and constantly being revised, but his emphasis on "less-informed" women as the vehicle of domestic disaster is telling.[14]

These warnings carried weight in part because women's experience-based practices were continually undercut by technological changes that added new variables to known procedures. For instance, one historic preserving method commonly known as open kettle required just a large saucepan in which sugared fruits (not vegetables) were brought to boiling, then poured into a hot, clean container and covered with glass, metal, wax, cloth, or even paper dipped in egg white or whisky (fig. 6.7). The seal was not necessarily airtight, but the method was most often used for jams and preserves, whose high sugar and acid content inhibited microbial growth. These imperfect seals also reduced the activity of *C. botulinum* spores, which create toxins in low-oxygen, low-acid, low-salt, low-competition, moist, room-temperature environments (Centers for Disease

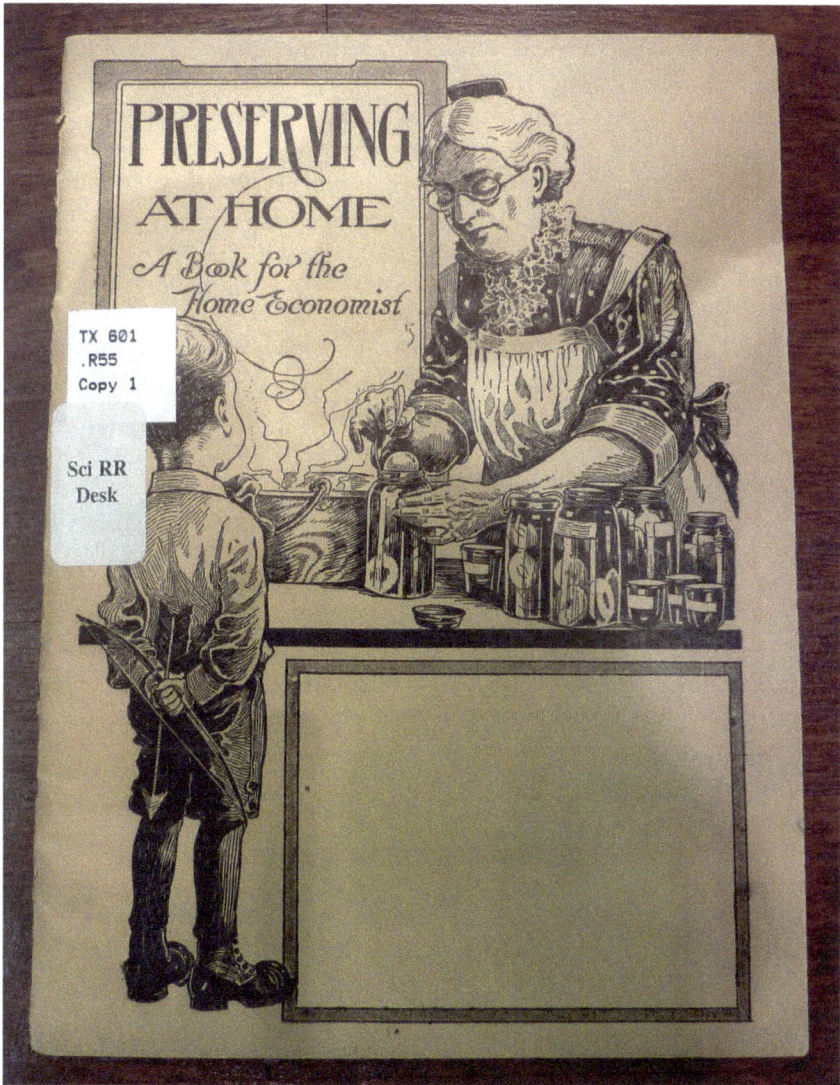

Fig. 6.7. This instruction manual features a white-haired matron demonstrating the "open-kettle" process, soon to be displaced by cold-pack processing. Riesenberg, Emily. 1916. *Preserving at Home: A Book for the Home Economist.* Chicago: Rand McNally.

Control and Prevention 1998). As hermetic seals improved in the early decades of the twentieth century and people began bottling low-acid vegetables and meats in addition to fruits, the "cold pack" (aka "cooked-in-the-jar") method was developed and recommended by scores of United States Department of Agriculture home demonstration agents and other experts. In this procedure, clean produce and meats were packed in clean hot jars, covered with hot syrup or brine, sealed, and immersed in a boiling water bath, with longer boiling times required for vegetables and meats. After it became known that botulism spores could survive in low-acid, low-oxygen preparations unless they had been heated above boiling (to 240° F) for a sufficient time, steam-pressure canners were recommended for most home bottling ventures (Andress and Kuhn 1988).[15] With improved designs, more affordable prices, and cooperative ownership, pressure canners (often called pressure cookers in vernacular speech) came into more common everyday use in the 1930s.

In this official instructional discourse, new directives undercut ordinary women's claims to expertise but rarely acknowledged that new technology (such as truly air-tight sealing compounds) or other contextual changes contributed to processing failures. The 1990 Kerr home canning manual, for example, simply headlines one section with the imperative "Forget Grandma's Open Kettle" (Kerr Glass Manufacturing Corporation 1990, 9). Transcribed accounts of canning in the twentieth century, however, reveal that many senior women have been both conversant in professional discourses and defenders of inherited tried-and-true strategies that remained successful in specific contexts. In these interviews, they display both their experiential knowledge and their familiarity with procedures recommended by credentialed experts. As they rehearse their shifting histories of practice, they drop in official terms and detail exact procedures, yet they also push back against the idea that their own mothers' knowledge was entirely and fatally flawed (fig. 6.8).

For instance, when interviewed at the turn of the twenty-first century, Mary Louis Evans of Clark County, Kentucky, recalled precisely how her family canned green beans without a pressure canner. In a recorded interview, she emphasized color, temperature, sanitation, specific measurements and cooking times, and visual check for a good seal. Her family would snap the strings off fresh clean beans the night before they were meant to be canned. Then, she said,

> You just heated the green beans until they lost that real bright green and they were hot through. And then you filled your jars. The jars had to be washed with soap and water and rinsed and kept hot. And so did the lids. Everything had to be clean and very hot. Or they wouldn't, didn't keep well.
>
> And then you filled the jar, we usually used quart jars, with the hot green beans and the liquid and added a teaspoon of salt for each quart.
>
> And then you put the tops on to seal them and put them in a boiling water bath and they had to cook for three hours.
>
> And then you took those out and let them cool. Checked to be sure they were sealed. And by then you were ready to start another batch. (Van Willigen and Van Willigen 2006, 215)

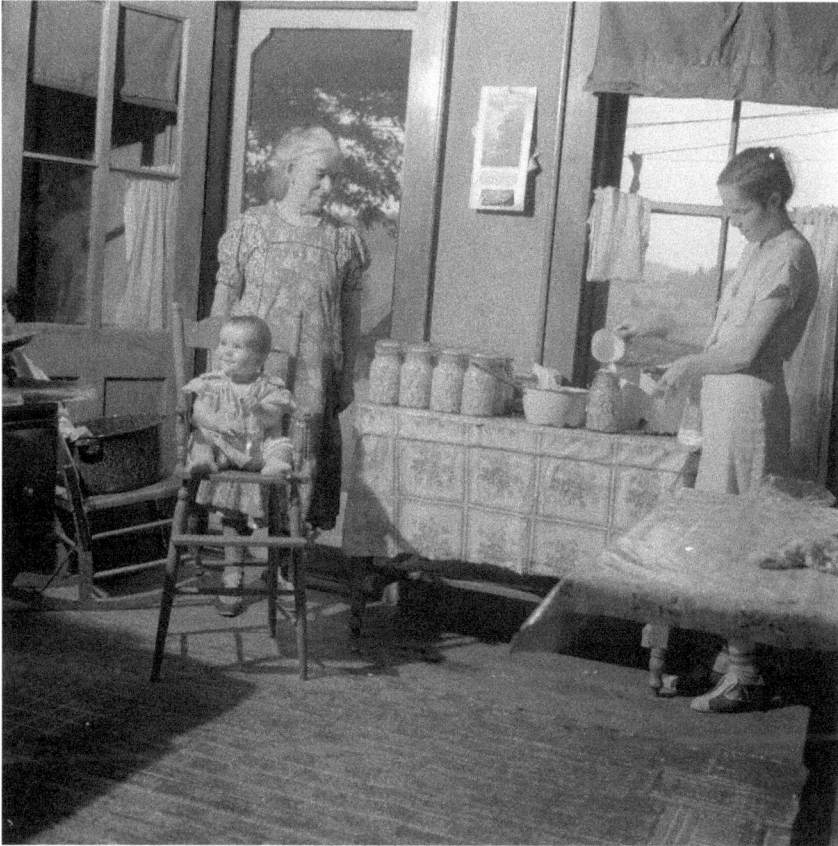

Fig. 6.8. Three generations participate in the preservation process. *Canning Beans in Farm Kitchen near Bristol, Vermont. Photograph by Louise Rosskam, July 1940. FSA/OWI Collection, Prints and Photographs Division, Library of Congress, Washington, DC. LC-USF34-012747-E.*

Evans's family usually did three batches of beans, with seven quarts per batch. Tomatoes, she recounted, must be scalded and peeled, then put in jars "with the juice. And they did not have to be processed nearly as long because they were so acid that they kept well. I think maybe twenty-five minutes for seven quarts sounds about right. And there again, you had to add the salt." She explained how to blanch corn before freezing it in order to arrest the action of enzymes. And she matter-of-factly mentioned her family's transition to newer technology when it became available: "Course by then we were using pressure cookers. Which I think it takes twenty-five minutes at ten pounds pressure for green beans. But by the time you get your pressure up to the proper point and then let it cool down afterwards so you can release them, it still takes a long time to can your beans" (Van Willigen and Van Willigen 2006, 216). Thus, Mary Louis Evans could rattle off the time and sustained pressure setting for a specific food using a pressure canner, but she also qualified her satisfaction with that process, suggesting that modern methods do not address all difficulties.

When asked about her family's canning, Hattie Wells (Harlan County, Kentucky) began by demonstrating her knowledge of disease agents, as well as her suspicion of industrial manufacturers and their recommendations for canning safely. Her mother, she said, "canned everything open kettle. And you know, today you pressure everything, and I wonder how we kept from gettin botchery [botulism] back then. And being real, real sick. But she canned everything open kettle. And they had some sort of an acid that they put in their corn and their beans to preserve them. And people used that. And I'm wonderin today if some of our cancer could have been caused by that acid."[16]

She goes on to trace the way her own family's practices changed over time. Yet she ends where she began, with the oldest practice—"open kettle"—and her mother's success using it:

> [In open-kettle canning, you just] put em in a dishpan and put em on and cook em for so long, and then put em in a can or a jar, and put some of that acid and seal em.
>
> But now, I remember my mother didn't have a pressure canner, but she got to where she put her beans in a jar and put them in a big black kettle and cooked em for three hours. Outside in the summertime. And, course that was cold packin or whatever you want to call it.
>
> And then of course her jams and jellies, she just made that open kettle on the stove. And she made plenty of them.[17] (Van Willigen and Van Willigen 2006, 213)

Ella V. Preston's family also canned outside (fig. 6.9). Describing the ways people processed peaches in Letcher County, Kentucky, she referenced her familiarity with three different processes: cold pack (in a boiling water bath), hot pack (in which foods are heated through before being enclosed in jars and subjected to the boiling water bath), and steam-pressure canning:

> They'd use a washtub and lay up a tin across the top of it, and build your fire on the outside.
>
> And they'd cold pack their peaches, or put em on the stove and heat em till you could get more in a can.
>
> And you'd put about nineteen quarts or half a gallon [half-gallon jars] in a washtub and build your fire underneath the washtub, have a fireplace and put your tin over top of it, and you got it boiling, it served as a pressure cooker [or rather, a water-bath boiler]. We got by with it. (Van Willigen and Van Willigen 2006, 214)

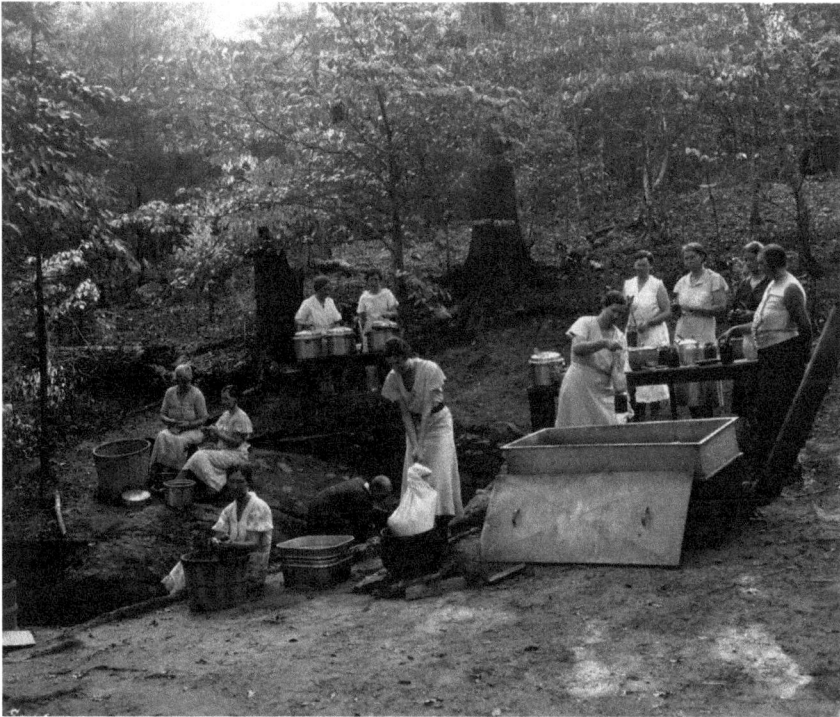

Fig. 6.9. An out-of-doors canning party, probably in western North Carolina, uses portable oil stoves to heat pressure canners. A large wood-fired boiling water bath processes high-acid fruits and vegetables. *USDA Extension Service, Miscellaneous American rural scenes, 1925-30, LOT 4777, Box 1 of 3. Prints and Photographs Division, Library of Congress, Washington, DC. S-18033-C.*

Her final statement dares the interviewer to question these methods and her own experience: "We got by with it."

A final example of a senior woman claiming lived expertise in relation to official discourse comes from Martha Arriola, a former ranch cook in Paradise Valley, Nevada. Arriola had emigrated from Germany in 1930 and spent most of that decade working for the William Stock outfit. When she changed employment in 1938, she left 1,280 half-gallon jars of food behind in the ranch's cellar, along with dried fruit, pickles, and blood sausage in crocks. Her reflections on canning meat show her awareness of approved methods, including knowledge she brought from Europe. "When the winter would get too strong, and they [the chickens] were too old," she remembered, "we canned maybe fifty at a time. We put them in jars, in a . . . big washtub," one large enough for the cowboys to bathe in. Like others who used washtubs to can in bulk, she set jars on hay placed in

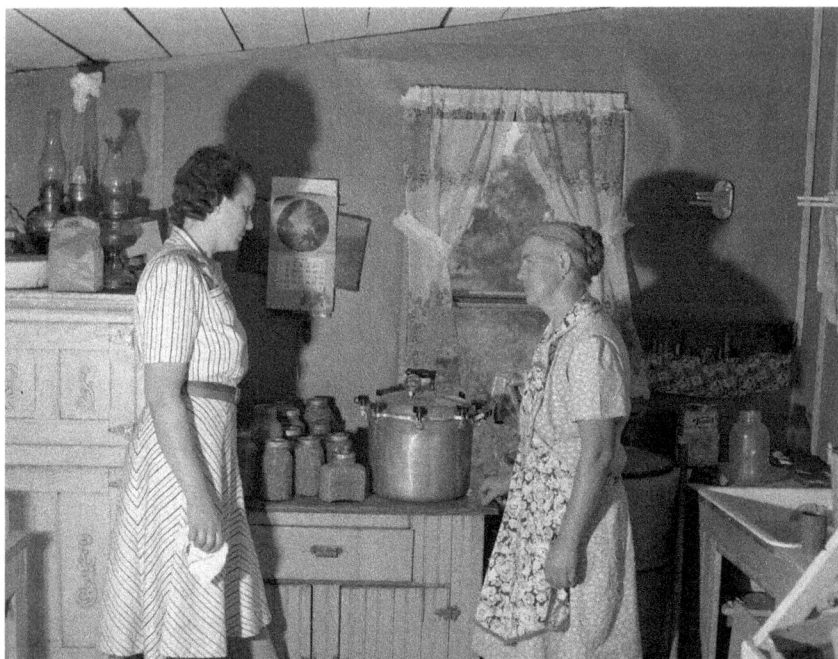

Fig. 6.10. *Wife of FSA (Farm Security Administration) Borrower Discussing Pressure Cooker with Home Supervisor. Photograph by John Vachon, Mille Lacs County, Minnesota, 1941. FSA/OWI Collection, Prints and Photographs Division, Library of Congress, Washington, DC. LC-USF34-063413-D.*

the metal bottom of the tub, which could hold at least thirty jars at a time. They boiled the submerged jars for three hours over the outdoor fire, then stored them in a brick cellar (Arriola 1978). Arriola knew about pressure canners and had used them (alongside water-bath boilers) at home in Germany. But the ranch didn't have a pressure canner, so "we canned it all in deep water, and it kept just as good—we never [laughing] had a poison case, or anything" (Arriola 1978).

In Ella Preston's case, the high-acid content of preserved peaches makes them very low risk with regard to botulism. But how could these Kentucky families have gotten away with processing low-acid green beans in a boiling water bath instead of the now-standard pressure canner? Perhaps the regional practice of boiling canned beans with pork or fatback before serving them also destroyed any toxin that may have developed during storage. Similarly, even though pressure canning is now universally recommended for processing low-acid meat—and most earlier recipes endorsed boiling bottles of meat for longer than three hours—something in the specific circumstances of processing and serving food

on the Nevada ranch staved off disaster. Food-borne disease is a complex phenomenon, and in the cases described above, any number of contextual factors
could have played a part in preventing illness.[18]

Broadly generalized instructions make sense for home canners today, because population mobility, climate shifts, innovative equipment, and new food
varieties result in ever-changing environments; with regard to botulism, relatively stable microcontexts are best when it comes to the application of experiential
knowledge. Yet those who have sought to guide home cooks toward ostensibly
safer (because more scientific) procedures have too rarely acknowledged the variable work processes, physical contexts, and technological systems in which human labor and biological life forms are embedded (Cowan 1983; cf. Tsing 2015).
As a result, situated logics of practice passed along by peers and elders may be
summarily discredited as ignorant or irrational (fig. 6.10).[19]

## Self-Reliance Is a Structural Issue

If lived experience can be dismissed as nothing more than old wives' tales, other
factors also diminish independence, interdependence, and material and intellec-
tual forms of productivity among older adults, particularly in rural areas. Seniors
living in "the country" are more at risk of experiencing food insecurity due to
lower incomes, higher food costs, narrower selection at stores, fewer public assistance programs, and inadequate transportation, especially when coupled with
a philosophical resistance to external aid (Quandt et al. 2001). The United States'
increasing reliance on an emergency network of food banks and food pantries,
rather than providing cash assistance, limits the choices of low-income individuals and isolates them from the broader social aspects of the consumer economy
(Dobson 2016).

Changes in material infrastructures alter participation in home food production as well. In Utah, for instance, nineteenth-century settlements were often
laid out with a central domestic nucleus surrounded by larger fields; individual
lots "in town" were explicitly large enough to accommodate a family garden,
small orchard, and a cow and chickens, and the community-regulated irrigation
system brought necessary water (fig. 6.11). These aspects of the built environment
encouraged Utah's strong food production and preservation culture. But in the
late 1970s, several ethnographers noted that rapid urbanization of the Wasatch
Front and the expansion of pressurized culinary drinking water systems had reduced lot sizes in the larger cities and disrupted irrigation schemes throughout
the state; in the more isolated towns, road improvements, access to grocery stores,
and shifts away from marginal farming lifestyles meant that home-based subsistence agriculture had declined dramatically, especially among younger residents.
By 1978, due to depopulation and little demand for land in less fertile areas, the

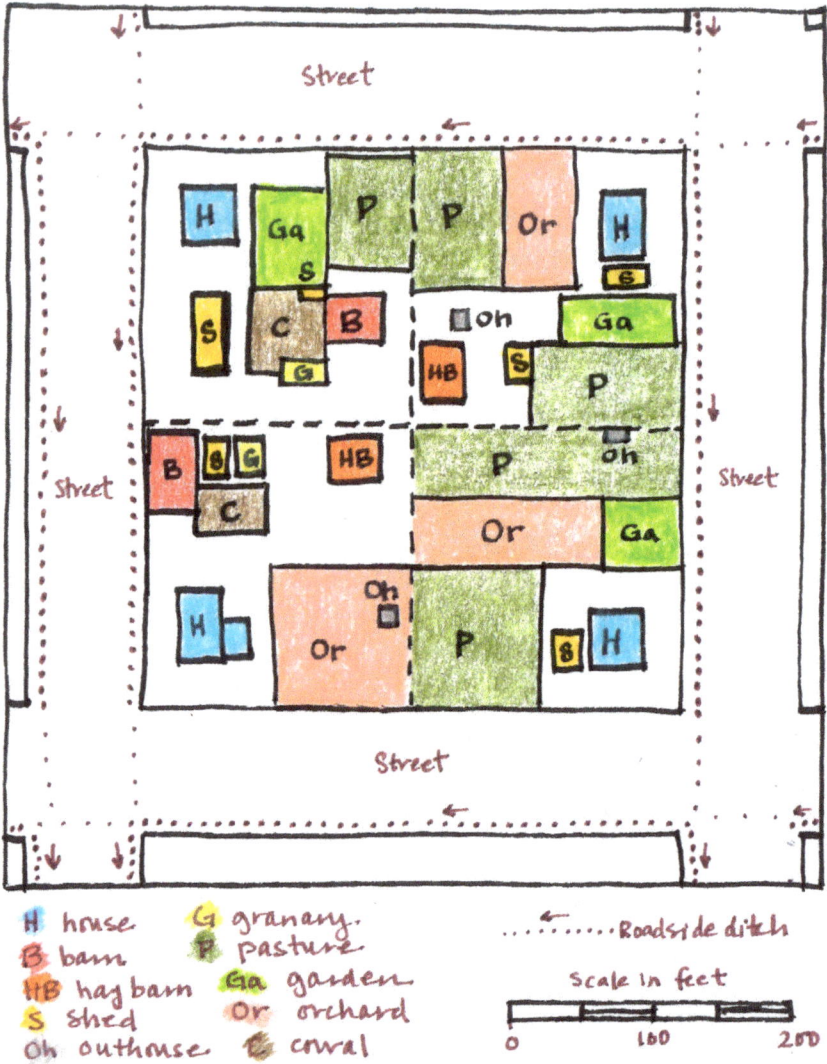

Fig. 6.11. A typical four-acre residential block in a small Utah town, showing a range of outbuildings as well as orchards, pastures, gardens, and corrals. Drawing adapted from an illustration by Richard V. Francaviglia, in *The Mormon Landscape* (New York: AMS Press, 1978), 17.

one-acre land parcels that characterized "Mormon village" settlements often included neglected orchards and "weed-infested lots in an uneasy conjunction with a garden, lawn, and home" (Francaviglia 1978, 28; Jackson 1978, 108; Nelson 1952).

Similar changes in population and degradation of public services continue to affect life elsewhere in rural America, due to the decline of coal, timber, and tobacco industries and the consolidation of family farms in pursuit of economies of scale. In the mid-1990s in West Virginia, (Warner) Howard Miller (b. 1918) explained how his family had "farmed the top of the mountain" in his youth: "We cut the trees down, and plowed up with a horse or dig it up, plant corn, potatoes, whatever." But now, he said, "People don't raise even a garden hardly. Very few of em has gardens around here" (H. Miller 1995, 2).

Even for those who want to continue to work in this way, systemic shifts make it difficult to acquire food production supplies. Instead of local manure, expensive inorganic fertilizers may need to be purchased; in addition, commercial (rather than heirloom or "saved") seeds can be costly and of questionable quality, and proprietary hybrid varieties must be purchased every year because they do not produce vigorous, "true" seed.

Changes associated with the life cycle also contribute to reduced participation in home-based food production. Of particular concern to seniors is poor health and reduced physical function. Almost three-quarters of the participants in Dobson's 2015 study had limited mobility. For instance, Gretta, age seventy-six, gardened until cancer made it too hard to walk to the garden and stay on her feet for long periods, while Terri found that her artificial knee and her husband's inability to run the tiller had minimized her family's ability to grow food (Dobson 2016, 72–73; Quandt et al. 2001). Aging partners or children who have left the nest also affect home food production, because motivation to garden has been linked to contexts in which coresidents can help to prepare ground, plant, harvest, cook, preserve, and eat food (Quandt 1994, 194).

## Still Working: Sustaining Traditional Forms of Food Productivity

Nationally, kitchen gardens are experiencing a comeback. According to a 2014 survey conducted by the National Gardening Association, between 2008 and 2013 household participation in food gardening (i.e., growing vegetables, fruits, berries, or herbs) across the United States increased 17 percent. Although those surveyed said that they were most interested in better-tasting and better-quality food, a majority were also concerned about economic uncertainty (participation in food gardening jumped 11 percent between 2008 and 2009, after the economy collapsed). Most recent food gardening in the United States has been associated with suburban, college-educated, middle-aged women, but the survey found substantial participation increases among millennials (aged eighteen to thirty-four,

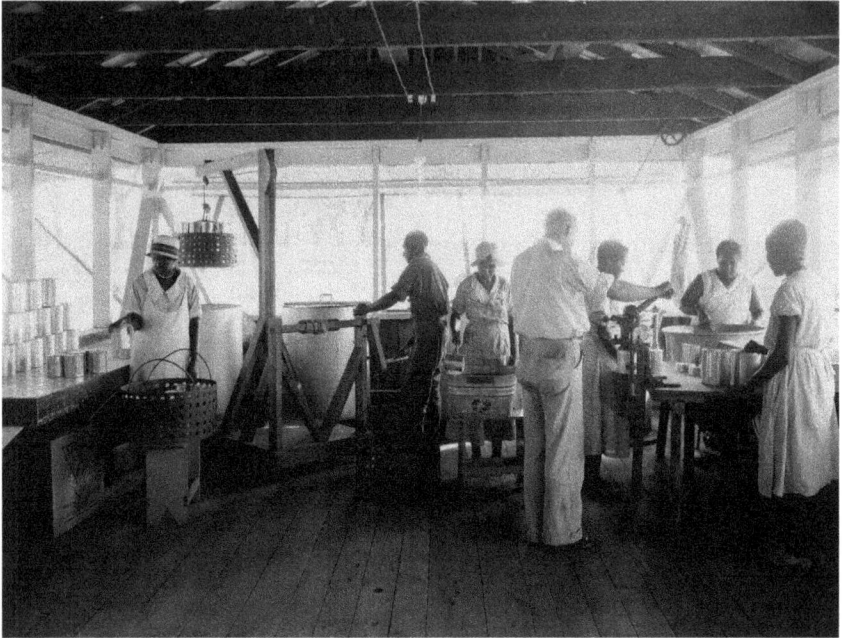

Fig. 6.12. Community canneries have existed in the United States since World War I, and a number of communities today still use World War II–era canneries or have established new ones. [*Preserving food in a community cannery.*] *USDA Extension Service, Miscellaneous American rural scenes, 1925–30, LOT 4777, Box 2 of 3. Prints and Photographs Division, Library of Congress, Washington, DC.*

including equal numbers of men and women), city dwellers, families with children, and those on the high (>$75,000) and low (<$35,000) ends of the income and educational spectrums (National Gardening Association 2014). At the same time, interest in home canning surged among these populations (Campoy 2009).

Given the mental, physical, and economic benefits of these activities, working to facilitate or recuperate them among older people in nonmetro areas makes sense. By 2050, one in four Americans will be sixty-five or older, and the ratio is even higher in rural areas: one in three (Berry and Glasgow 2013, 363). Among the latter population, the potential for apparent dependency is great. Rural seniors have less access to transportation, shopping, medical services, and social events; many also deal with physical limitations, restricted access to land or equipment, and real financial constraints (Dobson 2016; Quandt et al. 2001). These circumstances may interfere with traditional forms of productivity, further reducing material resources and frustrating identities grounded in the ideological and sensory pleasures of hard work, local foods, and neighborly support.

However, a number of nonprofit-sector organizations are attempting to intervene. In southwest Virginia, the Independence (VA) Farmers' Market, Mobile Food Pantry, and Grayson LandCare partnered to provide fifty EarthBox containers, soil, fertilizer, and seeds to elderly and low-income clients in 2014, and participants interviewed at the end of their second year with the project remained enthusiastic (Dobson 2016). Grow Appalachia, based at Berea College in Kentucky, partners with a range of community groups to offer garden grants, workshops, technical and physical assistance, and support for certified food processing kitchens in the southern mountains (Grow Appalachia 2017). Some elderly residents of central North Carolina, unable to garden themselves, rent or loan their land to others in exchange for a share of the produce. Communities in Utah have started similar practices that pair "resident" and "companion" gardeners (Quandt et al. 2001; Wasatch Community Gardens 2017). Sara Quandt and her colleagues have encouraged supporting community gardens and community canneries in order to create and allocate food surpluses in ways that align with local food ideologies (fig. 6.12); seniors may be more likely to seek out or accept food framed as "extra" or as a gift (Quandt 1994; Quandt et al. 2001). Finally, listening to and learning from elders who have pursued these activities all their lives acknowledges context-based mastery rather than dismissing old people's knowledge as dangerous, irrelevant, or simply outdated.

"Aging-in-place," write gerontologists Hellen Berry and Nina Glasgow (2013, 363), "is largely a function of how well individuals fit their environment both socially and physically." Assuming that aging and aged people are unproductive encourages dependence and isolation. But maintaining the larger material and social ecologies that support home food production and preservation can have multiple benefits. These practices maintain interpersonal networks of labor and exchange, demonstrate personal expertise and aesthetic taste, stimulate mental and physical activity, and offer material proof of continued productivity and relevance.

DANILLE ELISE CHRISTENSEN is Assistant Professor in the Department of Religion and Culture at Virginia Tech.

## Works Cited

Andress, Elizabeth L., and Gerald D. Kuhn. 1988. "Critical Review of Home Preservation Literature and Current Research." Athens: University of Georgia, Cooperative Extension Service. http://nchfp.uga.edu/publications/usda/review/report.html.
Antonucci, Toni C., Lisa Berkman, Axel Borsch-Supan, Laura L. Carstensen, Linda P. Fried, Frank F. Furstenberg, Dana Goldman, et al. 2016. "Society and the Individual

at the Dawn of the Twenty-First Century." In *Handbook of the Psychology of Aging*, 8th ed., edited by K. Warner Schaie and Sherry Willis, 41–62. San Diego: Elsevier Science.

Arriola, Martha. 1978. Interview by Suzi Jones, 1 August. AFC 1991/021 AFS#22725 (NV8-SJ-R22) Paradise Valley Collection (AFC 1991/021), American Folklife Center, Library of Congress, Washington, DC.

Arvin, Mildred. 2012. Interview by Chelsea Bicknell, 8 June. Folder 2, Box 1, Appalachian Foodways Oral History Collection (SAA 164), Berea College Special Collections & Archives, Berea, KY.

Baker, Lillie Liston to Ruth Elizabeth Baker Thompson, letters 1950–1960. MSS 1682 The Claude Vincent and Lillie Liston Baker Collection, Box 1, Folder 6, 20th Century Western & Mormon Americana, L. Tom Perry Special Collections, Harold B. Lee Library, Brigham Young University, Provo, UT.

Ball Brothers. n.d. (ca. 1905–1910). *The Correct Method for Preserving Fruit.* [Edition A1.] Ball Brothers Glass Manufacturing Company, Muncie, IN. Ball Corporation Collection 98.37, Box 1, Folder 1. The Minnetrista Heritage Collection, Muncie, IN.

Bateman, Mary Josephine Wilson. 1902–1905. *Mary W. Bateman Journal.* MS 10487, LDS Church History Library, Salt Lake City, UT. Microfilm.

Beaver, Patricia D. 1986. *Rural Community in the Appalachian South.* Lexington: University Press of Kentucky.

Berry, E. Hellen, and Nina Glasgow. 2013. "Conclusions and Policy Implications for Aging in Rural Places." In *Rural Aging in 21st-Century America*, edited by E. Hellen Berry and Nina Glasgow, 355–68. New York: Springer.

Bills, Gary E. 2012. Interview by Katherine N. Bills, 8 June. Folder 6, Box 1, Appalachian Foodways Oral History Collection (SAA 164), Berea College Special Collections & Archives, Berea, KY.

Blum, Marjorie. 2010. "The Pot Roast Story: A Leadership Tale." *Self-Defined Leadership*, August 31. http://selfdefinedleadership.com/blog/?p=158.

Brownlee, W. Elliot. 1979. "Household Values, Women's Work, and Economic Growth, 1800–1930." *The Journal of Economic History* 39 (1): 199–209.

Brunvand, Jan Harold. 1989. *Curses! Broiled Again!* New York: Norton.

Bryan, Leonard, and Mamie Lee Bryan. 1978. Interview by Pat Mullen, 6 September. Tapes AFS 21,585 (BR8-PM-R36) and AFS 21,586 (BR8-PM-R37), Blue Ridge Parkway Folklife Project (AFC 1982/009), American Folklife Center, Library of Congress, Washington, DC.

Campoy, Ana. 2009. "Putting Up Produce: Yes, You Can." *Wall Street Journal*, October 15. https://www.wsj.com/articles/SB10001424052748703787204574449160079437536.

Centers for Disease Control and Prevention. 1998. *Botulism in the United States, 1899–1996: Handbook for Epidemiologists, Clinicians, and Laboratory Workers.* Atlanta, GA: Centers for Disease Control and Prevention.

Certo. ca. 1951. "What Makes Jelly 'Jell'?" Undated booklet. Folder 11, Box 1, Series 1, Food Preservation and Home Canning Literature Collection, 1883–1980, Archives Center, National Museum of American History, Smithsonian Institution, Washington, DC.

Chaney, Arlene. 2012. Interview by Chelsea Bicknell, 21 June. Folder 10, Box 1, Appalachian Foodways Oral History Collection (SAA 164), Berea College Special Collections & Archives, Berea, KY.

Christensen, Danille Elise. 2015. "Simply Necessity? Agency and Aesthetics in Southern Home Canning." *Southern Cultures* 21 (1): 15–42.

Cohen, Gene D. 2006. "Research on Creativity and Aging: The Positive Impact of the Arts on Health and Illness." *Generations* 30 (1): 7–15.

Cowan, Ruth Schwartz. 1983. *More Work for Mother: The Ironies of Household Technology from the Open Hearth to the Microwave.* New York: Basic Books.

Cuddy, Amy J., Michael I. Norton, and Susan T. Fiske. 2005. "This Old Stereotype: The Pervasiveness and Persistence of the Elderly Stereotype." *Journal of Social Issues* 61 (2): 267–85.

DeVault, Marjorie L. 1991. *Feeding the Family: The Social Organization of Caring as Gendered Work.* Chicago: University of Chicago Press.

Dobson, Elizabeth R. 2016. "Case Study on a Container Gardening Program: Can Home Food Production Impact Community Food Security in Rural Appalachia?" Blacksburg: Virginia Polytechnic Institute and State University. https://vtechworks.lib .vt.edu/bitstream/handle/10919/71672/Dobson_ER_T_2016.pdf?sequence =1&isAllowed=y.

Entis, Phyllis. 2007. *Food Safety: Old Habits, New Perspectives.* Washington, DC: ASM Press.

Esposito, Joseph L. 1987. *The Obsolete Self: Philosophical Dimensions of Aging.* Berkeley: University of California Press.

Francaviglia, Richard V. 1978. *The Mormon Landscape: Existence, Creation, and Perception of a Unique Image in the American West.* New York: AMS Press.

Freidberg, Susanne. 2009. *Fresh: A Perishable History.* Cambridge, MA: Harvard University Press.

Grow Appalachia. 2017. *Grow Appalachia.* https://growappalachia.berea.edu/

Guest, David. N.d. "The Roast with the Ends Cut Off." *ActionCOACH.* Accessed March 12, 2016, https://www.actioncoach.com/The-Roast-With-The-Ends-Cut-Off?pressid=506.

Hall, Jacquelyn Dowd, James Leloudis, Robert Korstad, Mary Murphy, Lu Ann Jones, and Christopher B. Daly. 1987. *Like a Family: The Making of a Southern Cotton Mill World.* Chapel Hill: University of North Carolina Press.

Halperin, Rhoda H. 1990. *The Livelihood of Kin: Making Ends Meet "the Kentucky Way."* Austin: University of Texas Press.

Hannon, Kerry. 2015. "Is It Time to Abolish Mandatory Retirement?" *Forbes*, August 2. https://www.forbes.com/sites/nextavenue/2015/08/02/is-it-time-to-abolish -mandatory-retirement/.

Hatton, Clay. 2012. Interview by Chelsea Bicknell, 19 June. Folder 15, Box 1, Appalachian Foodways Oral History Collection (SAA 164), Berea College Special Collections & Archives, Berea, KY.

Higgins, Rita Rae. 2012. Interview with Katherine N. Bills, 2 July. Folder 17, Box 1, Appalachian Foodways Oral History Collection (SAA 164), Berea College Special Collections & Archives, Berea, KY.

Jabbour, Alan. 1981. "Some Thoughts from a Folk Cultural Perspective." In *Perspectives on Aging: Exploding the Myths*, edited by Priscilla W. Johnston, 139–49. Cambridge, MA: Ballinger.

Jackson, Richard H. 1978. "Religion and Landscape in the Mormon Cultural Region." In *Dimensions of Human Geography: Essays on Some Familiar and Neglected Themes*, edited by Karl W. Butzer, 100–27. Chicago: Department of Geography, University of Chicago.

Johnson, Colleen Leahy. 1983. "A Cultural Analysis of the Grandmother." *Research on Aging* 5 (4): 547–67.

Jones, Lu Ann. 2002. *Mama Learned Us to Work: Farm Women in the New South.* Chapel Hill: University of North Carolina Press.

Kerr Glass Manufacturing Corporation. 1990. *Kerr Kitchen Cookbook: Home Canning and Freezing Guide.* Los Angeles: Kerr Glass.

Kibbe, Madora. 2014. "The Pot Roast Principle." *Psychology Today*, February 8. http://www
.psychologytoday.com/blog/thinking-makes-it-so/201402/the-pot-roast-principle.

Kinnear, Dave. 2010. "The Roast Beef Story . . ." *Hire and Retain Top Talent*, February 3.
http://www.impacthiringsolutions.com/blog/the-roast-beef-story/.

Marsden, Michael T. 2010. "The County Fair as Celebration and Cultural Text." *The Journal of American Culture* 33 (1): 24–29.

McMillan, Reba, Clara Bell Valentine, and Euen Myers. "152. Bryan, Leonard Family."
2006. *Alleghany County Heritage*. Sparta, NC: Alleghany Historical and Genealogical Society.

Meyer, Madonna Harrington, ed. 2000. *Care Work: Gender, Labor, and the Welfare State*.
New York: Routledge.

Miller, [Warner] Howard, and Sadie [Ellis Cool] Miller. 1995. Interview by Mary Hufford,
22 April. Audio transcript, Folder 146, AFC 1999/008 SR108 (CRF-MH-A055), Coal
River Folklife Collection, American Folklife Center, Library of Congress, Washington, DC.

Miller, Sadie [Ellis Cool]. 1995. Interview by Mary Hufford, 28 September. Tape AFC
1999/008 SR123, Coal River Folklife Collection, American Folklife Center, Library of
Congress, Washington, DC.

Mikkelson, Barbara. 2005. "Grandma's Cooking Secret." *Snopes*, November 3. https://www
.snopes.com/fact-check/grandmas-cooking-secret/.

Morrow-Howell, Nancy, and Emily A. Greenfield. 2016. "Productive Engagement in Later
Life." In *Handbook of Aging and the Social Sciences*, 8th ed., edited by Linda George
and Kenneth Ferraro, 293–313. London: Elsevier Science.

Myerhoff, Barbara. 1992. "Aging and the Aged in Other Cultures: An Anthropological Perspective." In *Remembered Lives: The Work of Ritual, Storytelling, and Growing Older*,
edited by Mark Kaminksy, 101–26. Ann Arbor: University of Michigan Press, 1992.

National Center for Home Food Preservation. ca. 2001. "A Global Look at Some Home
Canning Activity Today." National Center for Home Food Preservation, University
of Georgia. http://nchfp.uga.edu/educators/natl_survey_summary.html.

National Gardening Association. 2014. *Garden to Table: A 5-Year Look at Food Gardening
in America*. South Burlington, VT: National Gardening Association. www.garden
.org.

Nelson, Lowry. 1952. *The Mormon Village: A Pattern and Technique of Land Settlement*.
Salt Lake City: University of Utah Press.

Parkin, Katherine J. 2006. *Food Is Love: Food Advertising and Gender Roles in Modern
America*. Philadelphia: University of Pennsylvania Press.

Prosterman, Leslie Mina. 1995. *Ordinary Life, Festival Days: Aesthetics in the Midwestern
County Fair*. Washington, DC: Smithsonian Institution Press.

Puckett, Anita. 2000. *Seldom Ask, Never Tell: Labor and Discourse in Appalachia*. New
York: Oxford University Press.

Quandt, Sara A. 1994. "Home Gardening and Food Preservation Practices of the Elderly in
Rural Kentucky." *Ecology of Food and Nutrition* 31 (3–4): 183–99.

Quandt, Sara A., Thomas A. Arcury, Juliana McDonald, Ronny A. Bell, and Mara Z.
Vitolins. 2001. "Meaning and Management of Food Security among Rural Elders."
*Journal of Applied Gerontology* 20 (3): 356–76.

Ramsay, Rose Moore. 2012. Interview by Chelsea Bicknell, 12 July. Folder 20, Box 1, Appalachian Foodways Oral History Collection (SAA 164), Berea College Special Collections & Archives, Berea, KY.

Roberts, Katherine R. 2006. "Storehouses of Abundance and Loss: Architecture, Narrative
and Memory in West Virginia." PhD diss., Indiana University, Bloomington.

Rockwell, Frederick Frye. 1918. *Save It for Winter: Modern Methods of Canning, Dehydrating, Preserving and Storing Vegetables and Fruit for Winter Use, with Comments on the Best Things to Grow for Saving, and When and How to Grow Them*. New York: Frederick A. Stokes.

Rowe, John W., and Robert L. Kahn. 1998. "Productivity in Old Age." In *Successful Aging*, 167–80. New York: Pantheon.

"Salicylic Acid as a Preservative." 1884. *Pacific Rural Press*, January 19, 51.

Sawin, Patricia. 2004. *Listening for a Life: A Dialogic Ethnography of Bessie Eldreth through Her Songs and Stories*. Logan: Utah State University Press.

Sayer, Liana C., Freedman, Vicki A., and Suzanne M. Bianchi. 2016. "Gender, Time Use, and Aging." In *Handbook of Aging and the Social Sciences*, 8th ed., edited by Linda George and Kenneth Ferraro, 163–80. London: Elsevier Science.

Severt, Carrie. 1978. Interview by Geraldine Johnson, 13 September. Tapes AFS 21,483 (BR8-GJ-R47) and AFS 21,484 (BR8-GJ-R48), Blue Ridge Parkway Folklife Project (AFC 1982/009), American Folklife Center, Library of Congress, Washington, DC.

Shuman, Amy. 2000. "Food Gifts: Ritual Exchange and the Production of Excess Meaning." *The Journal of American Folklore* 113 (450): 495–508.

Strasser, Susan. 1982. *Never Done: A History of American Housework*. New York: Pantheon Books.

Tanner, Fred W. 1935. "Home Canning and Public Health." *American Journal of Public Health and the Nation's Health* 25 (3): 301–13.

Tsing, Anna Lowenhaupt. 2015. *The Mushroom at the End of the World: On the Possibility of Life in Capitalist Ruins*. Princeton, NJ: Princeton University Press.

Utah-Idaho Sugar Company. 1950. "What Makes a Good Jar of Jelly." *Relief Society Magazine* 37 (9): back cover.

Vanek, Joann. 1979. "Time Spent in Housework." In *A Heritage of Her Own: Toward a New Social History of American Women*, edited by Nancy F. Cott and Elizabeth H. Pleck, 499–506. New York: Simon & Schuster.

Van Willigen, Anne, and John Van Willigen. 2006. *Food and Everyday Life on Kentucky Family Farms, 1920–1950*. Lexington: University Press of Kentucky.

Wang, Mo, and Junqi Shi. 2016. "Work, Retirement, and Aging." In *Handbook of the Psychology of Aging*, 8th ed., edited by K. Warner Schaie and Sherry Willis, 340–59. San Diego: Elsevier Science.

Wasatch Community Gardens. 2017. "Share a Yard." *Wasatch Community Gardens*. https://wasatchgardens.org/community-gardens/utah-yard-share.

# Notes

My sincere thanks to Rosemary Blieszner, Liza Dobson, Jon Kay, and two anonymous reviewers for their feedback on drafts of this article, and to archivists at the Alleghany County Public Library (Sparta, NC), American Folklife Center (Library of Congress), Berea College (Berea, KY), Brigham Young University (Provo, UT), the LDS Church History Library (Salt Lake City, UT), The Minnetrista Cultural Center (Muncie, IN), and The National Museum of American History for their assistance accessing primary source materials. This research was facilitated by a Gerald E. and Corinne L. Parsons Award, a Charles Redd Fellowship in Western American History, and a Kluge Fellowship.

1. The "doddering" perspective has more negative consequences in the paid workplace, as supervisors often assume that older workers are hopelessly outdated, unable or

unwilling to learn new skills, and thus unable to compete with younger cohorts (Wang and Shi 2016, 346).

2. While mandatory retirement has been illegal in the United States since 1986, when Congress added relevant language to the Age Discrimination in Employment Act, age limits are still common in some professional fields, are built into contractual agreements, or are informally enforced (Hannon 2015).

3. Interviews cited in this paper are drawn from archived transcripts or recordings that were accompanied by signed release forms. Liza Dobson's field consultants are identified by first name pseudonyms only.

4. For example, in their research on work, retirement, and aging, Mo Wang and Junqi Shi (2016, 339) explicitly define work as "paid employment activities."

5. Her effort in the garden had yielded other payoffs as well. Years earlier, when Chaney's daughter was working on her first batch of yeast bread for the fair, the girl had to keep punching down the dough because her mother was still tending to the garden and couldn't come help; in the end, the patiently worked bread won grand champion.

6. On the social value of work and self-sufficiency (especially well documented in the mountain South), see also Beaver 1986; Christensen 2015; Hall et al. 1987; Jones 2002; Sawin 2004.

7. Mountainous Grayson County averaged roughly thirty-five people per square mile in 2010; 19.1 percent of this population lived below the federal poverty line in 2014, compared to an 11.3 percent poverty rate in Virginia as a whole. The western part of the county, where Dobson did her research, had especially low food access, with many people living ten to twenty miles from the nearest grocery store. Two mobile food pantries served these communities; 65 percent of their clients were seniors who did not raise their own food due to physical limitations or lack of access to tools or soil. Dobson interviewed those who had participated in a free home container gardening program for two years. Most (thirteen out of sixteen) of those interviewed were women, and eight of them (average age, seventy-one) depended on social security benefits as their main source of income. All names from this study are pseudonyms (Dobson 2016).

8. *Truck* is a modification of *troquer*, the French term for *barter* (Freidberg 2009, 162).

9. For a discussion of intersections among excess, exchange, ideology, and social networks, see Amy Shuman's (2000) work on food gifts during Jewish celebrations of Purim.

10. Dorothy Noyes (1995, 457–58) identifies these contexts as those in which the frequency, duration, affective intensity, and material consequences of situated interactions are all very high.

11. Researchers have found that retirees benefit from sharing their knowledge with young people (Wang and Shi 2016, 354). While mental and physical functioning helps increase one's ability to offer goods and services to others, productivity also requires a belief in one's own efficacy—the development of a sense of mastery that comes from practicing one's craft in a social environment that offers confirming feedback (Rowe and Kahn 1998, 176).

12. Multiple factors influence microbial growth and the production of toxins in bottled foods, including altitude (because it affects boiling temperature); humidity; location (soil in some parts of the country contains more spores or different strains than others); container material (e.g., glass vs. metal), size, and condition; type of container seal; type of processing; condition of processing equipment (e.g., pressure gauges, depth of water bath); and the food's pH, maturity, microbial load, and density. Each factor is interrelated, and according to the Centers for Disease Control and Prevention (1998, 6), "changing one factor influences the effect of other factors." For instance, in the presence of specific proteins,

acid is less effective at inhibiting the production of toxins; furthermore, adding multiple ingredients to a food preparation can raise its pH level, making it less acidic. Some dense foods, such as mashed pumpkin, may create "low-acid pockets" that become dangerous. Boiling food after opening sealed jars—so that the temperature throughout is at least 185° F for five minutes—denatures botulism toxins that may have developed during storage.

13. While Jan Harold Brunvand's 1989 discussion of this narrative frames it as a "bungling bride" story, most recent interpretations focus on the follies of "slavishly" following tradition; Snopes.com, for instance, named the type "Grandma's Cooking Secret" (Brunvand 1989; Mikkelson 2005).

14. An early Ball Brothers "blue book"—*The Correct Method for Preserving Fruit*, published between 1905 and 1910—recommended a variety of methods for processing vegetables that are considered dangerous today. Lima beans and peas (both low-acid items) were supposed to be canned by adding cold water to filled jars, loosely covering with rubbers and tops, boiling them for three hours half-submerged in a deep covered pan, then reopening the jars and filling them to overflowing with boiling water before screwing down the tops once when hot and again when cold. Home processors at the turn of the century were directed to can corn, a vegetable notoriously hard to "keep" in a moist state, by boiling jars steadily for four hours and not reopening them afterward. High-acid tomatoes were processed open-kettle style: peeled and cooked with salt, then poured into glass jars, closed tightly, and turned upside down the next day (Ball Brothers n.d., 12–13). Even today, changes in the acidity of new plant hybrids, as well as other variables, regularly generate important new procedural recommendations by entities such as the University of Georgia–based National Center for Home Food Preservation.

15. *Clostridium botulinum* spores survive for six hours in rapidly boiling water (212° F), but just ten minutes at 240° F, a temperature that can only be achieved under pressure (Centers for Disease Control and Prevention 1998). Depending on the type and quantity of food being bottled, most contemporary recipes call for processing under pressure for longer than ten minutes.

16. In the late nineteenth century, salicylic acid and other chemicals were commonly used as food and beverage preservatives, although their safety was debated (Salicylic Acid 1884). They were also marketed for use in home canning.

17. Other interviews in which consultants specifically distinguish among different methods of canning include Arvin 2012, Bills 2012, and Ramsay 2012.

18. See note 12 for more on the ways relative humidity, regional soils, and postcanning cooking practices are related to the production and viability of toxins. For statistics on how many canners were using mixed and/or "not recommended" practices at the turn of the millennium, see National Center for Home Food Preservation ca. 2001.

19. The transfer of knowledge from very old to very young has sometimes been seen as evidence that practices are on the brink of extinction. But the adage that cultural practices "skip a generation" may simply reflect an established pattern of teaching and learning in which skills become "old time" simply because the teacher has returned to what was current during his or her own learning. In his work with elders skilled in various forms of traditional expression, folklorist Alan Jabbour observed that deeply rooted knowledge and embodied routines—such as fiddling—can persist despite physical infirmity or incongruent surroundings. "Expressive strain[s] . . . may lie fallow," yet are not extinguished (Jabbour 1981, 142). Jabbour suggested that gaps in practice have actually been the norm in many cultures: individuals learn skills as children, become proficient as young adults, move on to other concerns in middle age, yet turn to knowledge transfer in the last third of life.

# 7    Quilts and Aging

## Clare Luz and Marsha MacDowell

Contrary to common wisdom, not all quilters have been quilting for a lifetime.
Many start later in life, in response to an illness or difficult life event, then
discover that it's a tonic; a balm that satisfies multiple needs.

MacDowell, Luz, and Donaldson 2017, 106

QUILTMAKING IS A form of material culture production that scholars interested in the history and meaning of traditions in the everyday lives of individuals and communities have long documented and analyzed. Many studies have
explored the continuity of passing on skills and knowledge from one generation
to another or the use of this art form as a means of expressing life stories and
memories. Older quiltmakers are naturally apt to be the focus of such studies.
Yet, the prevalence of quiltmaking among elders begs deeper inquiry. What is the
connection of quiltmaking to the process of aging itself and why should we care?
Exploring these questions brings us face-to-face with the complex topics of aging
and mortality, and ways in which one can have the most optimal experience with
both. Most of us hope to enjoy a "good old age." For many, quiltmaking helps.

People of all ages engage in quiltmaking. Some do so to deal with the aging or death of loved ones, to cope with grief or anger. They also make quilts to
educate others and raise funds for research on illnesses including those more
common among older adults, such as Alzheimer's disease (fig. 7.1) and other de-
mentias (MacDowell, Luz, and Donaldson 2017). Here, we explore if there are
characteristics or a set of motivations among older quiltmakers that are unique
to advanced age or that one should consider when working with elders. We draw
heavily on stories told by or about older adults that link the quiltmakers' exper-

*The Expressive Lives of Elders* (2018): 138–152, DOI: 10.2979/expressivelivesofelders.0.0.08

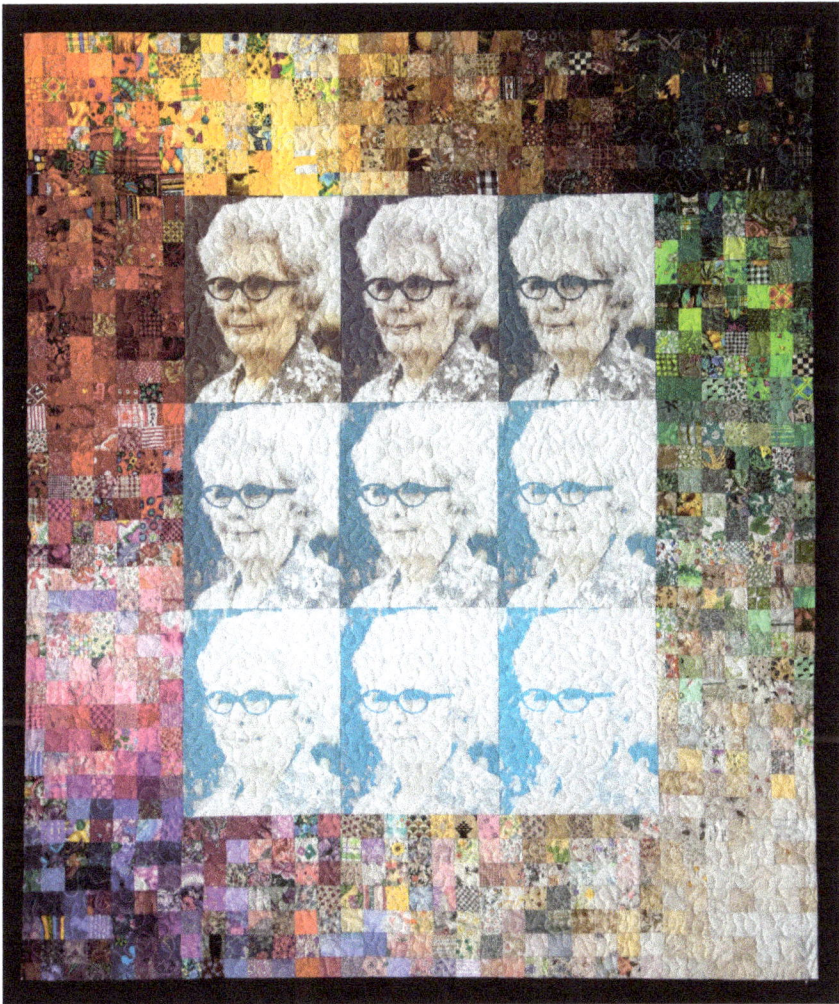

Fig. 7.1. Nevilyn, Linda J. Huff, Algonquin, Illinois, 2006. *Collection of Michigan State University Museum. Photograph by Pearl Yee Wong.*

ences related to aging and mortality with the material objects they create. As we will argue, our findings have relevance for all of us, personally and collectively. They mark a fledgling field of inquiry and invite others on a journey of discovery to understand more deeply the art of quiltmaking as experienced from the perspective of advanced age.

What is perhaps most instructive for those who work with elders is to have an appreciation for the length and breadth of their experiences, the universality of their core needs regardless of physical, mental, or cognitive status, and ways in which they choose to express their unique selves. For the elders showcased here, quiltmaking was the primary activity of choice. Each quilt is different, a creative expression that reflects a unique individual. All of the quiltmakers quilted because they drew immense pleasure in the quiltmaking itself. For many of them, the fact that they were helping others or others valued their quilts was added pleasure. It gave their lives meaning and purpose and was a vehicle for staying socially connected, even more so if they were sharing a sense of community with other makers.

Leona Scharfenberg, age ninety, provides an excellent example. When Leona moved into the Homestead at Hickory View Retirement Community in Washington, Missouri, she was disappointed to find that they didn't have a quilting group, so she decided to start one. She transformed her apartment into a gathering place for the Homestead Stitchers, a group of women ranging in age from seventy-five to ninety-five. They make and donate quilts to Grace's Place, an organization that offers no-cost childcare for families during a crisis. In the words of one group member, "It's volunteer work. It's just a way of living to do it. . . . That's what life is all about." Another said, "It feels really good. . . . There's satisfaction, and keeping busy and knowing you're doing something that's making a difference" (Butterfield 2013).

To understand how Leona's story connects to those of other elders and ultimately our own story, we need to step back and put this research in a larger context. The topic of folklore and the expressive lives of elders is both timely and important precisely because of recent and drastic demographic and social changes related to aging that will have an impact on everyone, both personally and collectively. We also need to examine the literature, see where there are major gaps, and begin to build a better knowledge base from which multiple disciplines can draw and work in collaboration with each other.

## Historical Context

Currently, the US population is rapidly aging, in part due to the swell of baby boomers who are now reaching age sixty-five at a rate of ten thousand per day (Fact Tank 2010). This trend will continue until 2030, and the social consequences will be dramatic for decades to come. The fastest growth is among the oldest old (aged eighty-five and over). The cumulative growth in the eighty-five-and-over population from 1995 to 2050 is anticipated to be more than 400 percent, and the proportion of that group in the total population is likely to increase from 1.4 percent in 1995 to 4.6 percent in 2050 (Ortman, Velkoff, and Hogan 2014). These demographic shifts affect all of us in extraordinarily personal ways as our parents, partners, and we ourselves age. They also affect us as a nation and as scholars.

When population aging occurs alongside other major shifts in the way we interact with and understand our world, new lines of inquiry emerge. It becomes ever more critical to examine the intersections of experience and knowledge, such as where the study of folk art and tradition crosses with that of gerontology, retirement, technology, social science, and medicine. For example, the Internet and social media have generated new forms of self-expression and relationships to one another, whether it be in the direction of engagement or anomie. We can no longer think of retirement as a single event that happens after years of loyalty to one employer. People are living longer, often with multiple careers that require new skills, and there is little fanfare when each job ends. Increased life expectancy also means a higher prevalence of people living with multiple, chronic, long-term conditions that affect the demand for supportive services, adaptable space, and new, creative ways to shape and protect a sense of identity. Moreover, there is now tremendous diversity among those we call elders, a group spanning four decades, so that concepts and theories that treat this massive group as one run the risk of being superficial at best.

Simultaneously, and in part as a result of these changes, there is a growing movement toward defining "good health" differently. The ramifications of a burgeoning population of older adults on healthcare costs has contributed to the promotion of healthy lifestyles to be sure, but more than this, people of all ages are recognizing the holistic nature of health. It is comprised of and affected by multiple aspects of ourselves: our spiritual, sexual, psychological, mental, and social selves. It is not just the absence of disease or illness but rather optimal functioning and quality of life regardless of our physical and other restraints. It is about what gives life meaning, what we value, and discovering how to live such a life.

This is not a new idea. People have long recognized that there is a universal need to feel that our life matters and that it is worth living. In writings throughout centuries about the "will to live," there seems to be a consensus that at its very core, it is composed of a sense of self-worth, a sense of purpose or feeling needed, identity, hope, futurity, social connectedness, and joy (Luz 2016). People of all ages need to be able to express who they are and have that expression affirmed by others. Variables such as health, culture, and economics may mediate forms of self-expression so that they change over time, but the critical components of what make a life worth living are ever present. In this context, the work of folklorists, gerontologists, artists, historians, educators, and others takes on new meaning. Listening to and affirming people's stories, expressed in multiple ways, is not merely interesting scholarship or best practice but an important contribution to sustaining life. In this way, the listeners become part of the story such as in the practice of "life review" through dialogue alone or through the making and describing of story objects, quilts, and other art forms. It has the power to actually change the story and the story's ending.

## Quilts and Health in the Scientific and Humanistic Literature

There have been limited systematic studies or recognition in the literature of the relationship between health and quiltmaking until recently. William R. Dunton Jr. (1946), a psychiatrist and quilt collector and considered the father of occupational therapy, wrote one of the earliest publications on quilt history in America. Dunton realized that "the process of selecting color and pattern, as well as the social interaction that quilts traditionally engendered, would be of great benefit to his 'nervous' patients. He thought his female patients could benefit from the quiet calming influence of needlework as well as the sense of accomplishment it brought" (Alexander 2012). However, the majority of subsequent studies related to health and the arts have focused on the therapeutic value of music, art therapy, writing, and movement. Moreover, in an extensive literature review conducted in 2010, researchers Heather Stuckey and Jeremy Nobel found that the vast majority of this literature is theoretical in nature without attention to measurable outcomes. It is only in the last ten years that the intersection of health and quilts in particular has emerged as an important topic worthy of systematic investigation.

As an example, more than six decades after Dunton's pioneering publication, Joshua Goh and Denise C. Park (2009) described one of the most rigorous studies to date to specifically include quiltmaking. Their randomized controlled intervention trial known as the Synapse Program was designed to evaluate the behavioral and neural impact of engagement in activities that facilitate successful cognitive function. Their work was based on the scaffolding theory of aging and cognition, which postulates compensatory changes take place in the brain to alleviate cognitive decline associated with aging and that this neuroplasticity can be experience dependent. One of the six control groups in the experiment was for individuals engaged in quiltmaking; another group engaged in digital photography. Quiltmaking and photography were chosen because they are deeply engaging tasks that could appeal to a broad spectrum of older adults, were complex enough to require learning new skills, and were fun. Research findings indicated that productive engagement caused a significant increase in episodic memory compared with receptive engagement (Goh and Park 2009).

Other quilt-focused studies now buttress these findings. Many are collecting data using sound research designs and validated instruments to measure coping, agency, well-being, and other outcomes. They are generating empirical data that can be used for multiple health-related goals such as for creating healing environments, therapeutic interventions, medical and public education, and fundraising (MacDowell, Luz, and Donaldson 2017). For example, anthropologist Virginia Dickie, who has specialized in geriatric occupational therapy, conducted a study with women quilters in North Carolina. She identified eight clusters of learning that take place while the women quilted and that such learning contributes to meaning and well-being. She also points out that according to an industry study, there are millions of quilters in the United States spending billions on their work. Therefore, quiltmaking is an occupation that is current, compelling, culturally relevant, and of economic interest (Dickie 2003). In our own research into the history of health-related quilts, we can say with confidence that millions of health-related quilts have been made, just in the United States alone (MacDowell, Luz, and Donaldson 2017).

## Quilts, Health, and Aging

Among the countless narratives of individuals for whom quilts figure centrally in their own health and well-being are a subset of those stories associated with older adults or elders, including those in their eighties and nineties—the oldest old—who are making quilts by the scores. These stories told by or about elders speak of how closely tied quiltmaking is to personal well-being. They also provide rich material for new understandings of the life experiences of elders and of contemporary expressive arts and cultural traditions. The impact of quiltmaking on vital life components—a sense of self-worth, a sense of purpose or feeling needed, identity, hope, futurity, social connectedness, and joy—was one of the central findings of the research on the relationship of quilts, health, and well-being we conducted with our colleague Beth Donaldson (fig. 7.2). Digging deeper into the stories of elders has led to a nascent understanding of how this relationship may play out differently among older adults. For example, although life review may happen at all ages, it perhaps takes on greater significance when done in old age. At that life stage, there is a longer life to look back on, a clearer awareness of one's mortality, different priorities, and the time to not only reflect on the events of one's life but also, importantly, to convey them to others in one form or another. Some quilts are made as a form of life review. Some are made as a way to express thoughts and feelings too deep for words. Among elders making quilts, it was most often a way in which they could establish a sense of purpose, identity, and connectedness to others and sidestep boredom by engaging in an activity they enjoyed.

As in all ages, most elders seek out ways to pass time that fit well with their individual functional ability, interests, and resources. They continue to have a vibrant desire to live fully in ways that express who they are—their history, values, personality, experiences, and talents. These desires are not so different from those of younger people; nor is the desire for dignity and respect. However, advancing age is marked by having to relinquish major sources for fulfilling core human needs, through a series of life events such as a final retirement, multiple chronic conditions and disabilities associated with physical aging, empty nests, and the deaths of family and close friends. As we live in a youth-centric, antiaging cul-

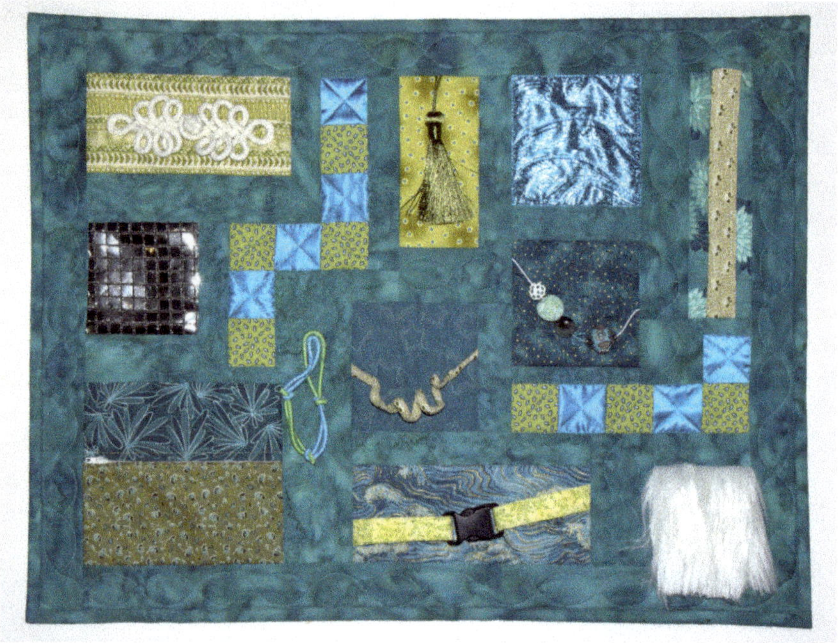

Fig. 7.2. Fidget Quilt, Beth Donaldson, Lansing, Michigan. *Collection of Beth Donaldson. Photograph by Pearl Yee Wong.*

ture in which individual identities are often tied to paid work, these losses and connections to others can be difficult to replace.

Fortunately, advancing age also brings new and positive resources from which to draw: resilience, a bank of skills and experience, a longer worldview, a greater appreciation for life viewed in the context of a closer proximity to death. Awareness of mortality can sharpen the idea that "life is short" and shift priorities such that the need to lead a meaningful, enjoyable life may become more acute. Add to this that the ending of key roles and obligations can mean that there is finally time to engage in activities, old or new, that are personally rewarding. A growing body of literature confirms that if the fit is good, quiltmaking is a powerful way to meet multiple needs unique to older adults, thus contributing to a more positive aging experience. The individual stories told here represent the fact that whether they are lifelong or novice quilters, many elders find ways to engage in this creative art form and in so doing, provide celebratory examples of what is possible as we age.

Everett Drevs's story provides just such an example. Drevs came to quilt-making later in life. A retired community college biology teacher of Estherville,

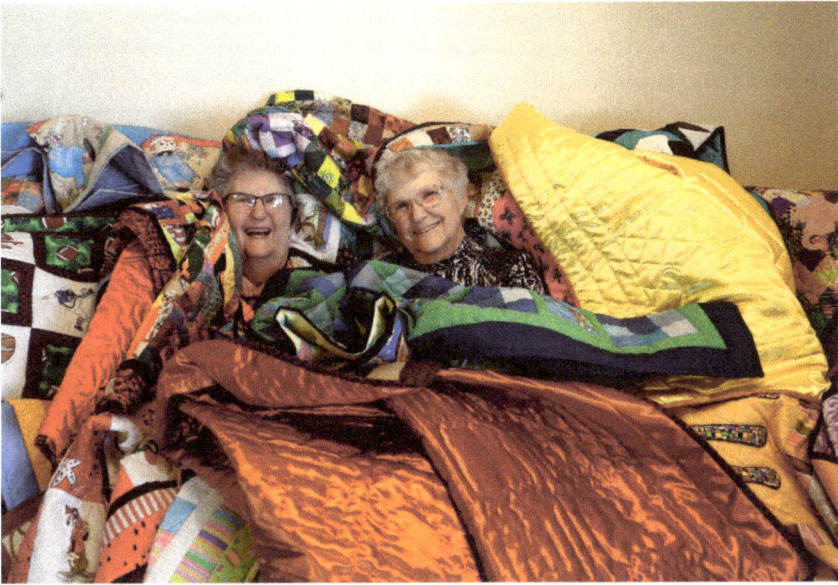

Fig. 7.3. Sisters and octogenarians Joyce Lynn and Joann Bentz in a pile of some of the more than one thousand quilts they have made. *Photograph by Ilene Olson. Courtesy of* Powell *(Wyoming)* Tribune.

Iowa, he learned quilting from his wife, Teddy, in 1996 when she was diagnosed with non-Hodgkin's lymphoma and he was diagnosed with prostate cancer. Using fabric left by his mother and grandmother as well as the clothing of Teddy after she passed away, Drevs took up sewing and found it relaxing. He is now an avid quilter and a member of the local North Star quilt guild, which makes quilts for local hospice patients. Drevs also makes them for hospice patients on his own, because they helped his wife in her last days (Kilen 2014).

Likewise, sisters Joyce Lynn and Joann Bentz of Powell, Wyoming, took up serious quiltmaking later in life as a way to engage in service work to benefit the community (fig. 7.3). In 2005, then aged seventy-five and seventy-three, respectively, they started a project to make "a few quilts" and send them to St. Jude's Research Hospital to comfort children who were being treated for cancer. But they soon found that, as Bentz said, "Once you get started, you just can't quit," and in eleven years, they made more than a thousand quilts. The sisters cut, piece, add batting to, and machine quilt fabric that they embroider by machine; they keep their embroidery machines running, with the aid of computerized designs, for six to eight hours per day (Olsen 2015). In a 2016 phone conversation with the sisters, they reported that they had made at least an additional thousand quilts since Olsen's article that they gave to many other individuals and organizations. The pleasure that these quiltmakers receive from quiltmaking is increased by knowing they are helping others through their craft.

Also inspired by being able to make a meaningful difference in other people's lives, Marie Bryant, age seventy-one, recalled the day she delivered her quilting group's quilts to nursing home residents in Franklin County, Virginia. "The staff told me about this one woman who never got out of bed, so I left her quilt for last," she said. Bryant assured the elderly woman that the quilt was free, and she picked one out. "I went back to the nurses' station and I turned around, and there she was, out of her room," Bryant said. For members of the Red Hill Baptist Quilters, founded by Bryant in 1989, quilts offer comforts both tangible and intangible (Adams 2013).

Countless stories can be found of elders who have been lifelong quiltmakers and are now using their love of quilting to help others. There is Eva Bossenberger who, at a hundred years old, wakes up early most mornings and goes straight to the sewing machine to sew dresses for little girls that will be packed and sent in a shoebox as part of a ministry called Operation Christmas Child sponsored by Samaritan's Purse (2017). And Trudie Hughes, who retired from running a quilt shop, now works seven days a week, ten hours per day, making sixty quilts a month that she donates to La Causa in Milwaukee, Wisconsin, a safe haven for children. She does it for "fun." In her words: "It's just something that I absolutely love to do. The nicest part is that you are able to donate your time and materials to someone who really appreciates it. Until I fall over, dead, I will keep quilting" (Morris 2017). Like Trudi, Hilda Wanner, an eighty-eight-year-old resident of a retirement community in Fargo, North Dakota, has been making quilts for thirty years. Over a two-year period, she made and donated forty quilts to new patients at the Roger Maris Cancer Center. She sums up her reasons by saying, "I feel like I am doing something worthwhile. If it is a comfort to them, it is a comfort to me. . . . One thing I can say is that I am never bored" (Wallevand 2016).

These particular elders aren't quiltmaking as a hobby for part-time recreation. They are almost driven by their passion to engage in something they love doing for the benefit or recognition of others. It brings meaning to their lives. For some, old age has given them the gift of time that they didn't have in their younger years. Irene Dahlen, age eighty-eight from Breckenridge, Minnesota, now sews nonstop and has been dubbed the "Quilting Warrior." She has donated as many as one hundred quilt tops in one year to Grace Lutheran Church, which sends finished quilts to Lutheran World Relief and the Orphan Grain Train, both humanitarian organizations with volunteers working around the world. In her words: "I always felt guilty that I couldn't be helping more, so now I've tried to make up for it" (McDermott 2017). Iris Young, age ninety-seven from Nebraska, explains that she did not learn how to quilt until she retired from being an el-

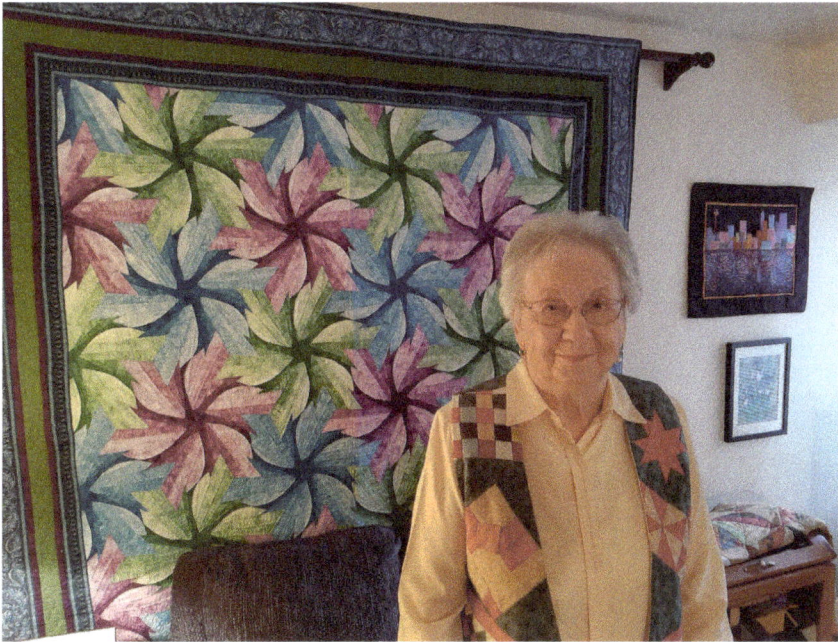

Fig. 7.4. Iris Young. *Photograph by Jessica Hoppe. Courtesy of ThurstonTalk.com.*

ementary school teacher and had the time (fig. 7.4). It was something to fill her days but quickly turned into a passion that has lasted seventeen years. She simply says, "I do it because I love it, and the kids appreciate it" (Hoppe 2017).

There are elders who clearly have mortality in mind when they make a quilt, in anticipation of their own death as well as that of others. The director of nursing in a nursing home in Grand Rapids, Michigan, tells the story of a resident one day asking why it is that new residents come in through the front door while those who die are taken out the back door, without any acknowledgment or ceremony. The resident shared the difficulty of not knowing what has happened to someone and not being able to mark the passing or honor the person's life in a dignified manner. The nurse agreed and advocated for a change in policy; people who died would be taken out the front door and the residents and staff would have the opportunity to recognize their life. An idea developed to make quilts to cover the person as they left the facility. Over time, these quilts, many made by the residents themselves, became more personalized, and eventually, residents began making quilts for themselves in anticipation of their own death, using familiar fabrics and favorite colors. This story speaks of the power of a simple quilt to humanize an otherwise sterile, impersonal procedure.[1] This practice of

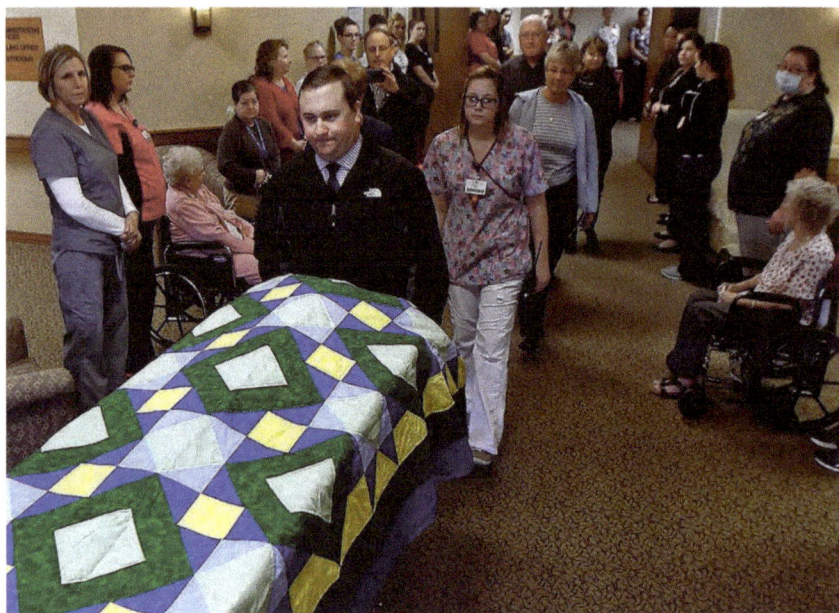

Fig. 7.5. Luther Acres staff line a hallway for a farewell Walk of Honor. *Photograph by Chris Knight. Courtesy of LNP Correspondent.*

using what are sometimes called dignity quilts is appearing more often across the country. Luther Acres retirement community in Lititz, Pennsylvania, now holds "walks of honor" for residents who have died (fig. 7.5). Employees and others line the sides of the hallways and pay tribute as a body, covered by a colorful handmade quilt, is ushered out of the facility by the funeral director (Hawkes 2017). The Pinetree Patchworkers in Brainerd, Minnesota, donate dignity quilts to local nursing homes and funeral directors. Their goal is to show honor and respect to people who have died and bring comfort to grieving families and staff. As one quiltmaker stated, "When people think of a quilt, they think of warmth and home" (Anon. 2004).

For some who come to quiltmaking in middle age, the connection to a community of people through quilting and feeling like a member of that community becomes important to healing, well-being, and quality of life and will ultimately sustain them into their old age. This speaks to the potential of quiltmaking to serve as a protective resource, one that can be nurtured over time and strengthen one's ability to adapt to life losses and changes associated with aging and more advanced age. As an example, Ruth A. White of Ithaca, New York, is a member of the Tompkins County Quilters Guild and a self-described "cancer fighter." In a newspaper article by Joanne Hindman (2015), she reported to have "discov-

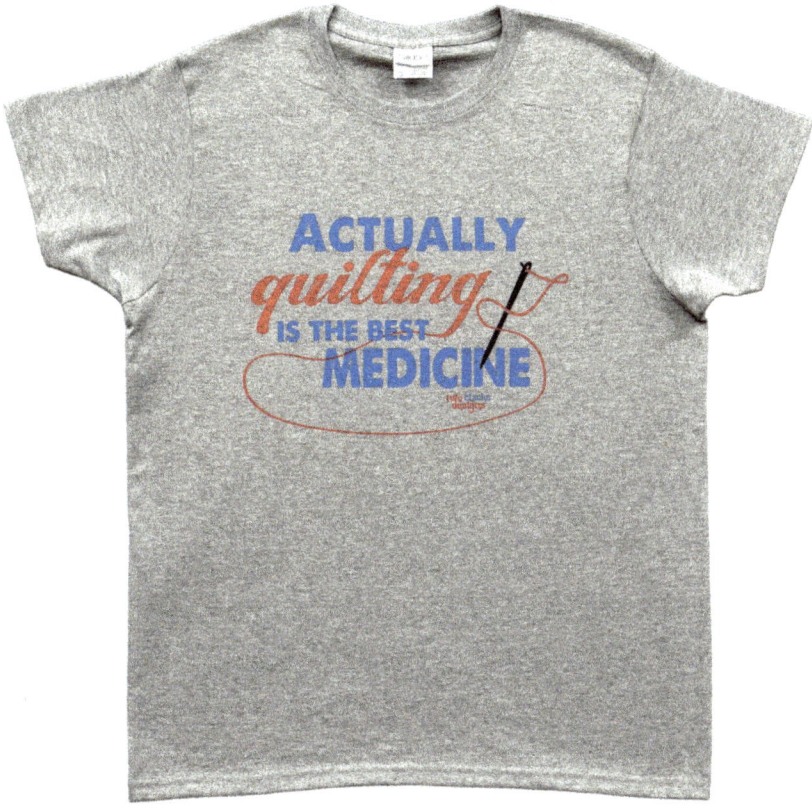

Fig. 7.6. T-shirt. *Collection of Michigan State University Museum, purchased from Two Chicks Design.*

ered the therapeutic value of quilting almost as soon as she joined a quilting group while working in College Station, Texas in her early forties. The traditional work bees that her Texas quilt group organized freed her to talk about and work through personal issues, particularly her depression and loneliness. 'The camaraderie around quilters, talking through our issues together,' she says, 'worked better than the drugs!'" Since that time, nearly two decades have passed, and she refers to other members of the guild to which she belongs as her "sisters-by-choice."[2] These relationships will surely have a positive impact on the quality of her aging experience.

In each of the above stories—all associated with older adults, including many among the oldest old—we hear words that reflect characteristics of well-being. These are people in later years who do not convey boredom or helplessness. Ruth White's case suggests that quiltmaking could be considered in earlier years as a proactive agent of positive aging. Whether they were lifelong quiltmakers or relatively new to the craft, these individuals tell vibrant stories of quiltmaking, which provides them with a clear sense of identity, purpose, and connectedness to others. They proclaim that they make quilts because "it is fun." It provides a profound sense of agency and makes them feel good to help others. Frances Reynolds states, illness can become a "master status" in a person's life, cutting them off from their usual sources of self-identity and self-esteem. Textile art can become an avenue for challenging this status and managing illness (Reynolds 1997; Reynolds and Prior 2003). Perhaps the same could be said for aging. In a society that intrinsically promotes a youth-oriented, antiaging bias, elders can become cut off from their usual sources of identity, recreation, and social connectedness. Quiltmaking can become an avenue for challenging and celebrating aging.

## Summary

The humanistic and scientific literature is now verifying what many quiltmakers already know—the making of quilts is therapeutic (MacDowell, Luz, Donaldson 2017). The work is tangible, tactile evidence of progress toward recovery or of acceptance of living with altered conditions, of perseverance, of life-affirming activity, and of continuing to be productive in the face of adversity. We posit that systematic studies of the making and use of quilts as they relate to health and well-being has great potential to help us understand the human experience of illness and health, understand the place of traditional arts within these experiences, advance medical knowledge, and ultimately enhance the quality of health care, health outcomes, and even of life itself. They can also help us understand and enhance the experience of aging into advanced age. As more such studies are undertaken, we believe the empirical evidence will substantiate what we already believe to be true, that quiltmaking can equal good health and good aging and that, at least for some, "quilting is the best medicine" (fig. 7.6).

CLARE LUZ is Assistant Professor in Family Medicine at Michigan State University. A gerontologist, her research focuses on the direct care workforce and aging and the arts. She is coauthor (with Marsha MacDowell and Beth Donaldson) of *Quilts and Health* (IUP).

MARSHA MACDOWELL is Professor and Curator at the Michigan State University Museum as well as Director of the Quilt Index and the Michigan Traditional Arts Program. She is co-author (with Clare Luz and Beth Donaldson) of *Quilts and Health* (IUP).

## Works Cited

Adams, Duncan. 2013. "'A Token of Love,' Stitch by Stitch." *Roanoke Times*, October 7. http://www.roanoke.com/news/local/roanoke_county/a-token-of-love-stitch-by -stitch/article_b7083a9d-6308-51b6-8b09-a02a0da9ed86.html.

Alexander, Karen. 2012. "William R. Dunton (1868–1966), Quilt Collector, Author, Psychiatrist." *The Quilters Hall of Fame Blog*, January 16. http://thequiltershalloffame .blogspot.com/2012/01/william-r-dunton-1979-honoree.html.

Anon. 2004. "Local Quilters Present Dignity Quilts to Funeral Directors." *ECM Archives*, May 18, 2004. http://archives.ecmpublishers.com/2004/05/18/local-quilters-present -dignity-quilts-to-funeral-directors-2/.

Butterfield, Karen. 2013. "Homestead Stitchers Delight in Donating Handmade Quilts." *Missourian*, May 6. http://www.emissourian.com/features_people/senior_lifetimes /homestead-stitchers-delight-in-donating-handmade-quilts/article_e65d4713-70e6 -534b-ae3c-a28a4bb43522.html.

Dickie, Virginia Allen. 2003. "The Role of Learning in Quilt Making." *Journal of Occupational Science* 10: 120–29.

Dunton, William Rush Jr. 1946. *Old Quilts*. Baltimore: Privately printed.

Fact Tank. 2010. "Baby Boomers Retire." Pew Research Center, December 29. http://www .pewresearch.org/fact-tank/2010/12/29/baby-boomers-retire/.

Goh, Joshua O., and Denise C. Park. 2009. "Neuroplasticity and Cognitive Aging: The Scaffolding Theory of Aging and Cognition." *Restorative Neurology and Neuroscience* 27 (5): 391–403.

Hawkes, Jeff. 2017. "How Luther Acres Nursing Home Honors the End of Life by Not Shunning Death." *Lancaster Online*, March 2. http://lancasteronline.com/insider/how -luther-acres-nursing-home-honors-the-end-of-life/article_fc60cfb2-f92a-11e6-8204 -73ce2ec49b7e.html.

Hindman, Joanne. 2015. "Witness to Fatal Ithaca Crash Turns to Quilting after Trauma." *Ithaca Voice*, September 21. http://ithacavoice.com/2015/09/witness-to-fatal-ithaca -crash-turns-to-quilting-after-trauma.

Hoppe, Jessica. 2017. "97-Year-Old Breaks Age Barriers with Passion for Quilting." *Allpeoplequilt.com* (blog), October 24. http://www.allpeoplequilt.com/magazines -more/97-year-old-breaks-age-barriers-passion-quilting.

Kilen, Mike. 2014. "Widower's Quilts Piece Together Family Stories." *USA Today*, April 20. https://www.usatoday.com/story/news/nation/2014/04/20/widowers-quilts-piece -together-family-stories/7913757/.

Luz, Clare. 2016. "Family Medicine: Bridge to Life." *Journal of the American Board of Family Medicine* 29 (1): 161–64.

MacDowell, Marsha, Clare Luz, and Beth Donaldson. 2017. *Quilts and Health*. Bloomington: Indiana University Press.

McDermott, Carrie. 2017. "86-Year-Old Breckenridge Woman Made 100 Quilt Tops in 2016." *Daily News*, January 13. http://www.wahpetondailynews.com/news/year-old -breckenridge-woman-made-quilt-tops-in/article_597866da-d9a3-11e6-a3b6 -8f18e72701ed.html.

Morris, Paul. 2017. "This Retired Grandma Spends 10 Hours a Day Making Quilts. What She Does with Them? Beautiful!" *Little Things* (blog), September 5. https://www .littlethings.com/grandmother-quilts-work-inspire/.

Olsen, Ilene. 2015. "Quilting Sisters: 1,000-Quilt Goal Reached." *Powell Tribune*, December 29. http://www.powelltribune.com/news/item/14370-quilting-sisters-1-000-quilt -goal-reached.

Ortman, Jennifer M., Victoria A. Velkoff, and Howard Hogan. 2014. "An Aging Nation: The Older Population in the United States." *Population Estimates and Projections Report* (May): 1–28. https://www.census.gov/prod/2014pubs/p25-1140.pdf.

Reynolds, Frances. 1997. "Coping with Chronic Illness and Disability through Creative Needlecraft." *British Journal of Occupational Therapy* 60 (8): 352–56.

Reynolds, Frances, and Sarah Prior. 2003. "'A Lifestyle Coat-Hanger': A Phenomenological Study of the Meanings of Artwork for Women Coping with Chronic Illness and Disability." *Disability and Rehabilitation* 25 (14): 785–94.

Samaritan's Purse. 2017. "100-Year-Old Seamstress Makes Dresses to Pack in Shoebox Gifts." *Samaritan's Purse* (blog), August 25. https://www.samaritanspurse.org/article/100-year-old-seamstress-makes-dresses-to-pack-in-shoebox-gifts/.

Stuckey Heather L., and Jeremy Nobel. 2010. "The Connection between Art, Healing, and Public Health: A Review of Current Literature. Framing Health Matters." *American Journal of Public Health* 100: 254–63.

Wallevand, Kevin. 2016. "Sewing Has Helped One 88-Year-Old's Mind Stay Sharp while also Helping Local Cancer Patients." WDAY-TV, June 27. http://www.wday.com/news/4063389-sewing-has-helped-one-88-year-olds-min d-stay-sharp-while-also-helping-local-cancer.

## Notes

1. Field notes from meeting with staff at Pilgrim Manor Retirement Community, Grand Rapids, Michigan, January 26, 2011.

2. Ruth White, artist statement, submitted to Beth Donaldson, Clare Luz, and Marsha MacDowell, March 15, 2016.

# 8  Curating Time's Body

## *Elders as Stewards of Historical Sensibility*

### Mary Hufford

In the 1980s, folklorists were rethinking the implications of our field's historical reliance on the elderly. Insights emerging from the field of gerontology affirmed what we had long sensed, that there was much more to be gained from engaging the long memories of seniors than the "study of culture at a distance" (Mead and Metraux 1953). As the remarkable infrastructure for the support of folk arts spread across the states, enabling the growth of public folklore, a pattern explored by essays in the present volume was gaining clarity. At a certain point as we grow older, many of us discover a need to give form to memory, through practices of remembering, suturing together parts of a life lived long over far-flung times and places. Whether these practices take the form of folk art as officially recognized, the imperative, its means of expression, and its effects are now widely recognized. What we may be slower to appreciate is how much skin we, the researchers, have in this game.

Marjorie Hunt, Steve Zeitlin, and I wrote about this pattern, in which we saw a promising and exciting new direction for age-related folklore research and public programming. The book we coauthored, *The Grand Generation: Memory, Mastery, Legacy*, was inspired in part by anthropologist Barbara Myerhoff's pioneering ethnography of a community of elderly Jews in Venice, California, *Number Our Days*. In the film of the same title, Myerhoff avows her personal stake in that research: "Someday, I'm going to be a little old Jewish lady." Tragically, that didn't happen. Myerhoff died at the age of fifty, leaving us to reflect upon—with growing appreciation for—the wisdom suffusing her ethnography of elderhood. Rapidly advancing toward elderhood in our own families and communities, in

*The Expressive Lives of Elders* (2018): 153–171, DOI: 10.2979/expressivelivesofelders.0.0.09

recent years we've experienced in visceral ways the accumulating effects of our participation in what Barbara Kirshenblatt-Gimblett, in her introduction to *The Grand Generation*, called the "recurrent and enduring" aspects of life, given form, made into artistic objects of reflection, sometimes by people closest to us.

Over the three decades since we coauthored *The Grand Generation* as thirty-somethings-only Steve Zeitlin had children at that time—we have all three been through the cycle of childbearing and rearing. For me, those experiences have illuminated something that one of the featured artists, Ethel Mohamed, expressed so eloquently—the strange sense of déjà vu from a new point of view granted by a different role in the same process, seen first through our eyes as children, then through our eyes as parents. "I am the age of whoever I'm with," she says in the film *The Grand Generation*.

Our implication in these cycles can catch us by surprise. When my mother, Barbara Hufford, took up carving in her sixties, I realized I was becoming the *daughter* of a folk artist (fig. 8.1). From the mid-1990s until her death at the age of 87 in 2017, Barbara produced and gave away dozens of carvings commemorating events and scenes of our extended family life—my brother's home improvement projects (fig. 8.2), my sister's interest in lepidoptera (fig. 8.3), my husband's woodworking (fig. 8.4), the burrowing owls that shared the neighborhood in Cape Coral (fig. 8.5). Her carvings consoled us for the deaths of cherished pets (figs. 8.6 and 8.7). Barbara's choice of materials represented the ecological settings in which she and my father lived out their later years—the eastern deciduous woodlands, the bayous of Louisiana, the beaches and canals of southwest Florida, and the pine-covered piedmont of Richmond, Virginia. Her creations of acorn caps (fig. 8.8), seashells (fig. 8.9), pine needles (fig. 8.10), and gourds she grew in her garden (fig. 8.11) populate the homes of children, nieces, nephews, neighbors, and grandchildren.

For a family reunion when they lived in Florida, Barbara made twenty canes out of the flower stalks of coconut palms, each topped with a figure she thought would be meaningful to the recipient (fig. 8.12). Everywhere my parents walked during the last few years of their lives, their canes accompanied them. While helping to care for my mother following my father's death, I witnessed firsthand a principle emphasized in *The Grand Generation*: the prompting of sociality through folk art. As we walked through my mother's neighborhood, down the hallways of her church, from parking lots to grocery stores, and along park trails, we were accosted by strangers marveling at her cane (figs. 8.13–8.15). Conversations happened—frequently.

In 2012, Barbara was featured in an exhibit at the Ward Museum on Maryland's Eastern Shore, curated by Cindy Byrd, a graduate of the Penn Folklore program. Inspired by my mother's carvings displayed at our home in Bala Cynwyd, Byrd developed the exhibition titled, "Making Her Mark: A Showcase of Women Carvers."

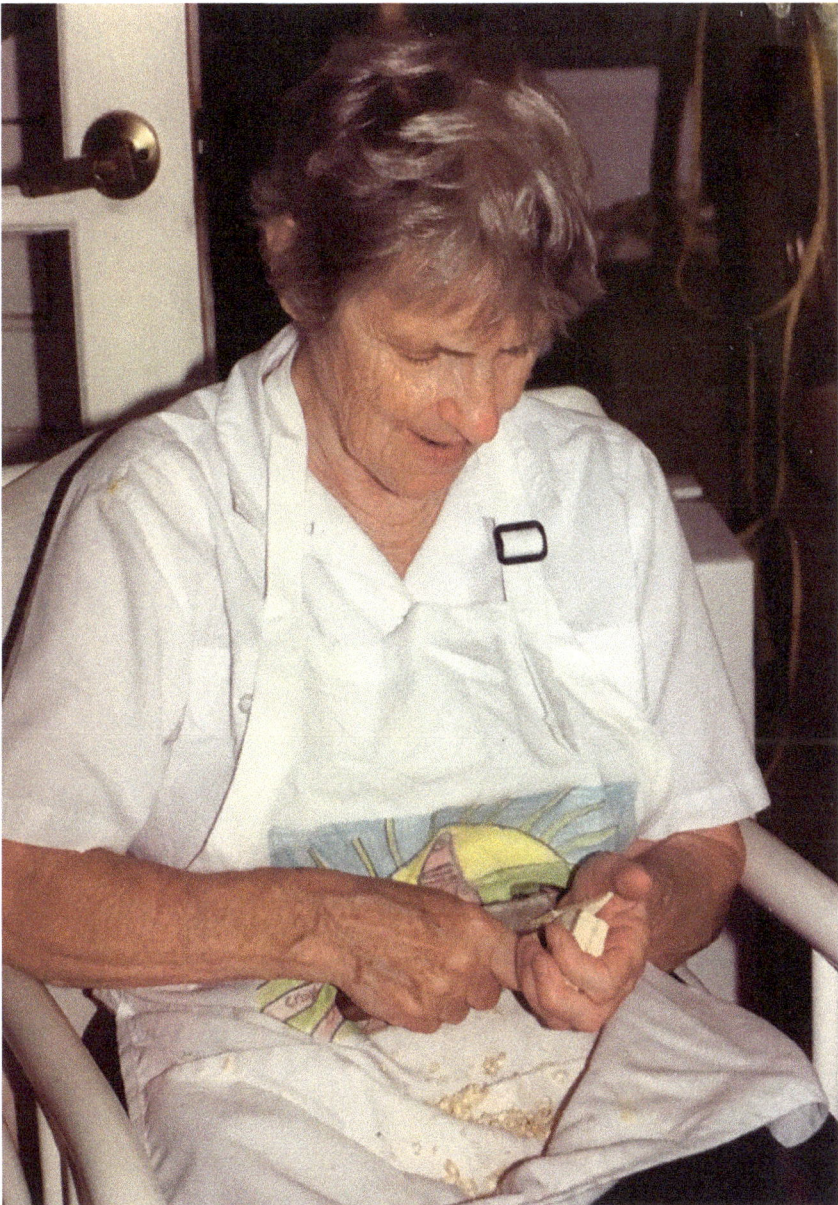

Fig. 8.1. Barbara Hufford, carving in the early 1990s, Cape Coral, Florida. *Photograph by Mary Hufford.*

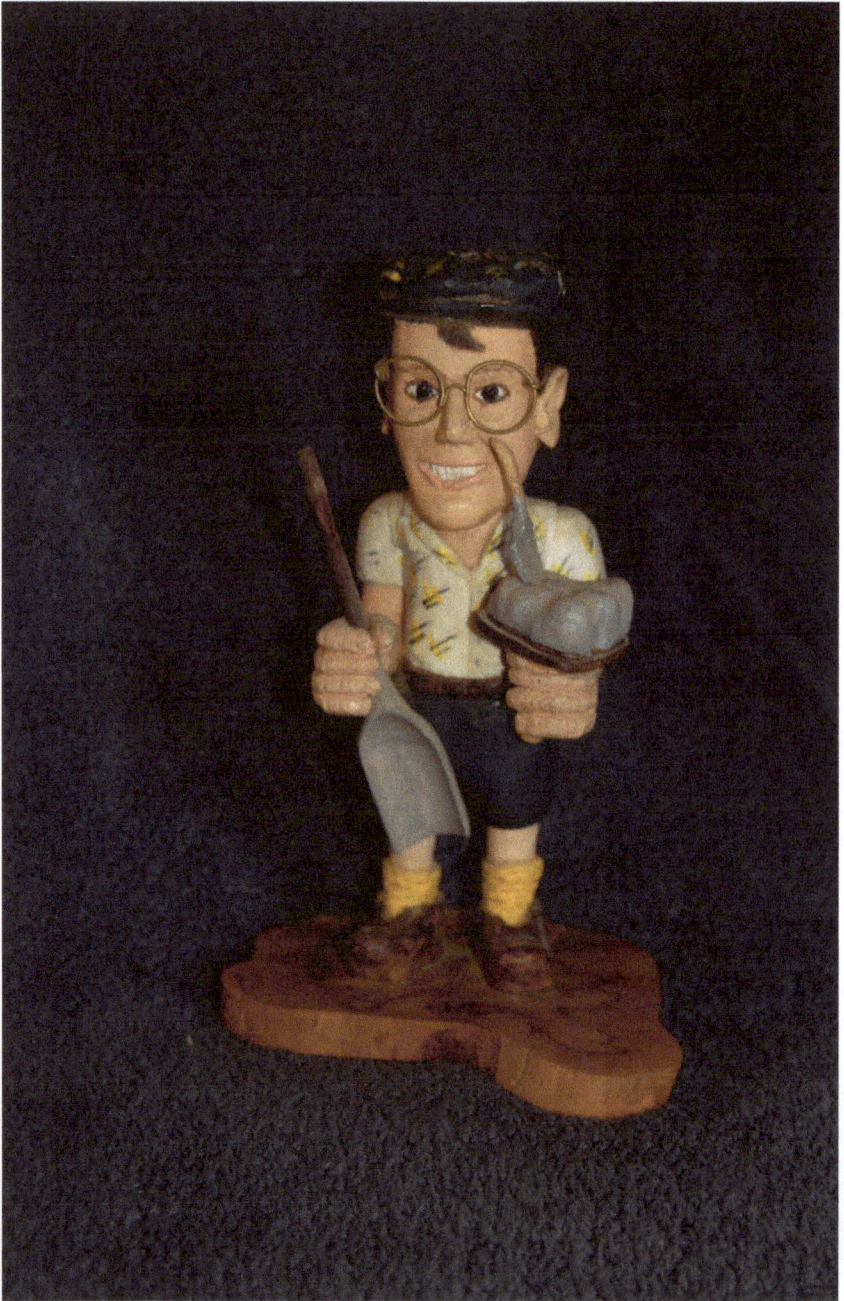

Fig. 8.2. Barbara's oldest son, Duane. *Photograph by Mary Hufford.*

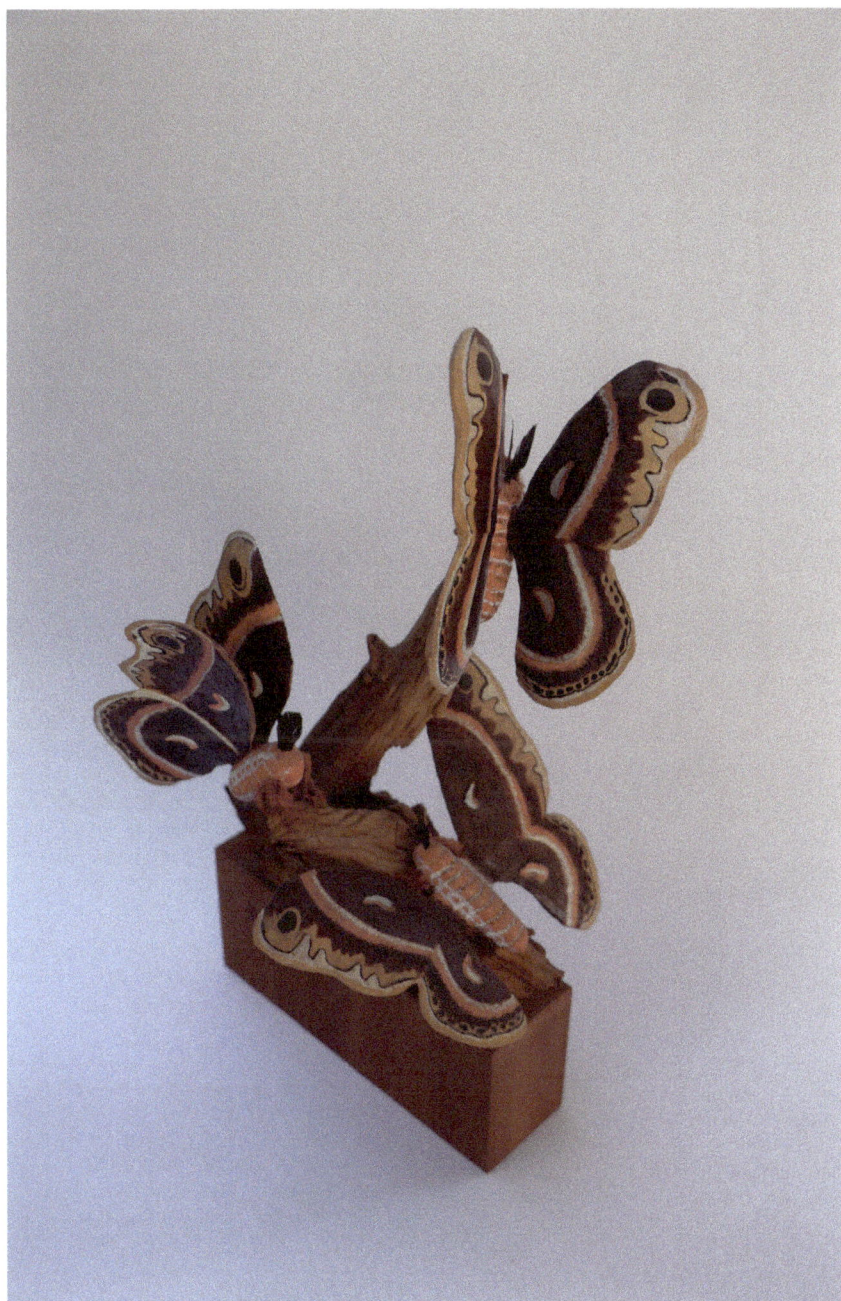

Fig. 8.3. Cecropia moths that Barbara raised with her children in Delmont, Pennsylvania, and that her children continued to raise with their children. *Photograph by Mary Hufford.*

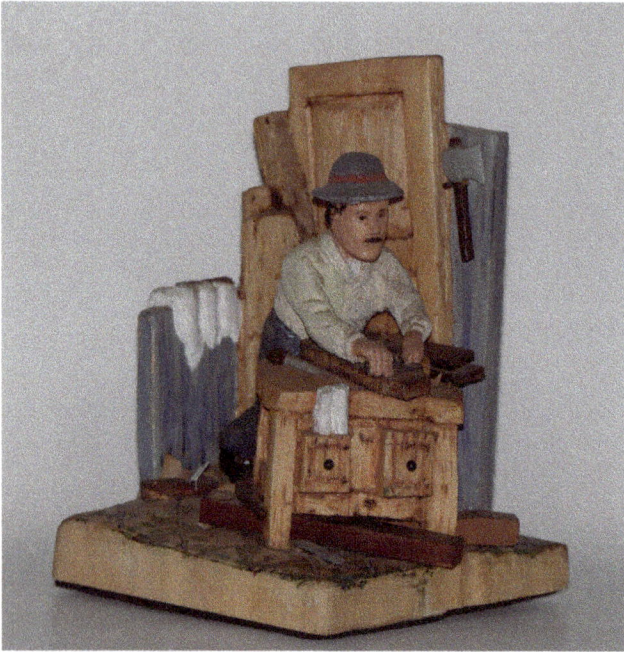

Fig. 8.4. Barbara's son-in-law, Steven Oaks, a woodworker, who provided Barbara with scraps from his shop for her to carve. *Photograph by Katherine Oaks.*

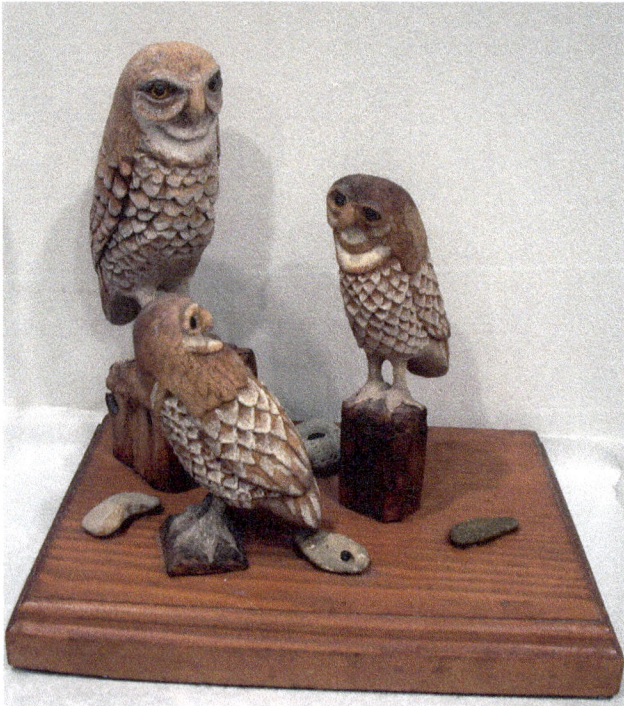

Fig. 8.5. Burrowing owls, a protected species that lived in Barbara's neighborhood in Cape Coral, Florida. *Photograph by Rosanne Healy.*

Figs 8.6 and 8.7. Barbara's carvings commemorated cherished pets of her grandchildren: Alice, a guinea pig, and Jackson, a golden retriever (whose favorite toy was a stuffed lady bug). *Photographs by Katherine Oaks.*

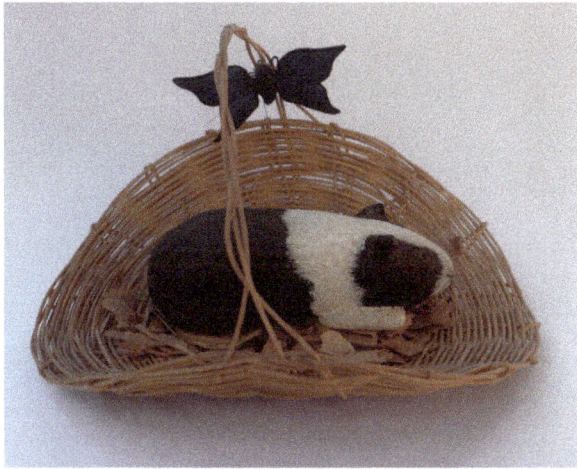

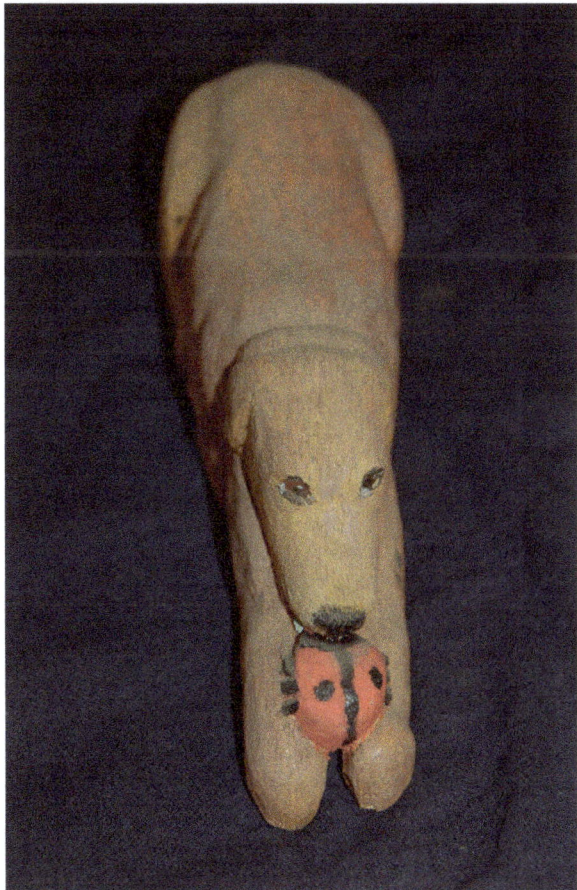

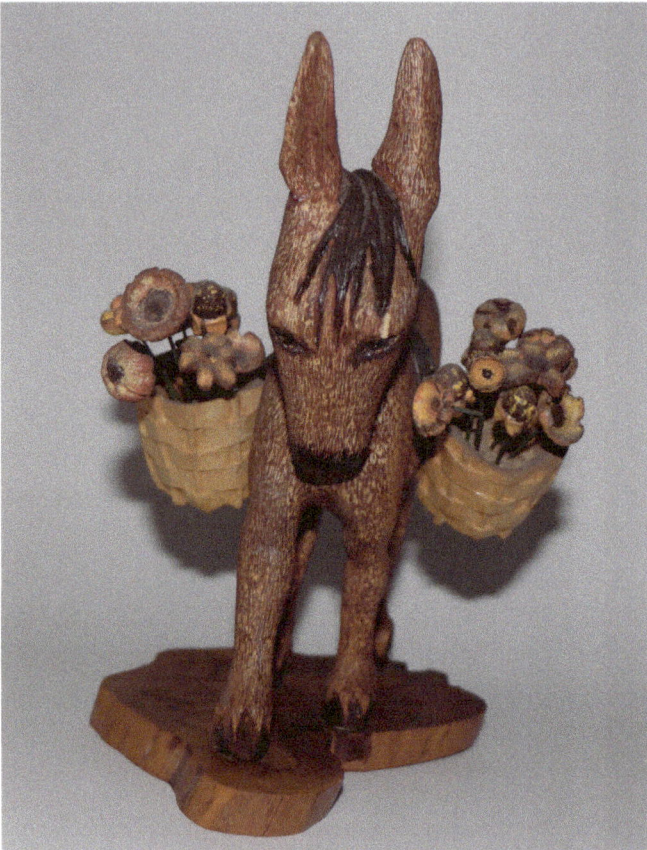

Fig. 8.8. A burro, carved by Barbara for her granddaughter. The carved wooden baskets are filled with flowers made from acorns picked up on a walk Barbara took with her granddaughter. *Photograph by Katherine Oaks.*

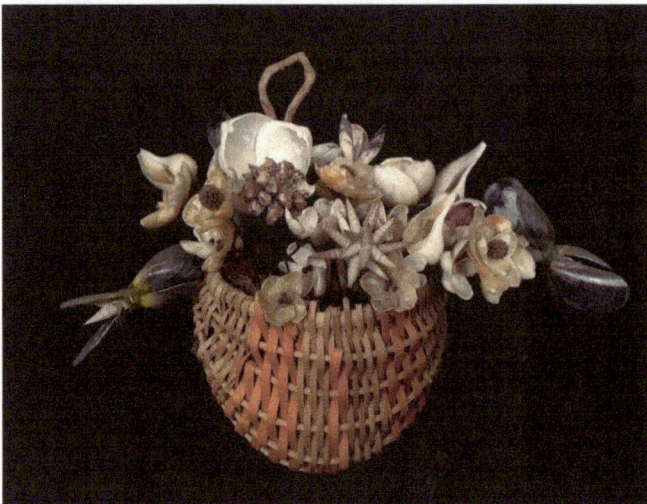

Fig. 8.9. Flowers made from seashells collected on Sanibel Island. Barbara made the basket using gnarled driftwood for a handle. *Photograph by Mary Hufford.*

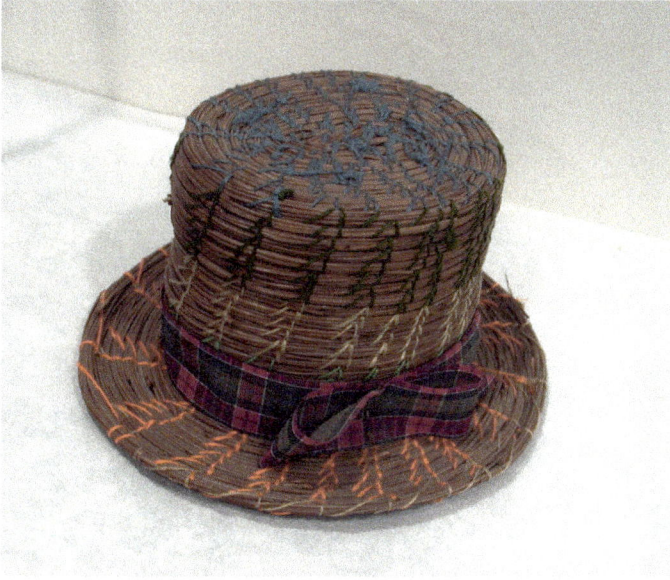

Fig. 8.10. Top hat made from long-needle pine needles that Barbara collected from her backyard in Richmond, Virginia. *Photograph by Rosanne Healy.*

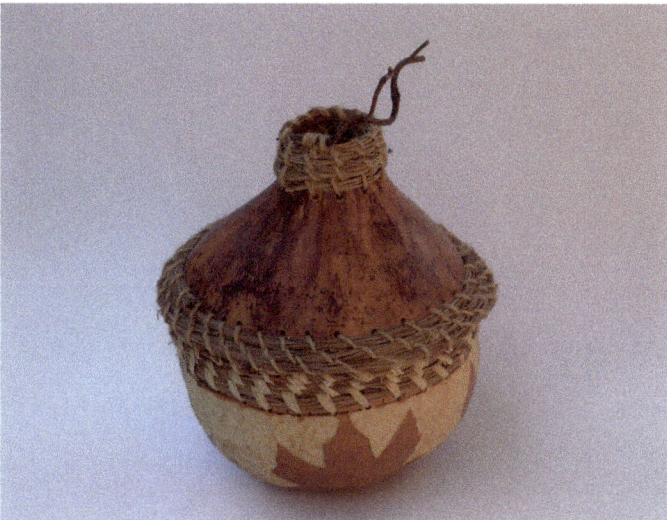

Fig. 8.11. Lidded gourd container trimmed with long-needle pine. The gourds were grown in the garden in Richmond. *Photograph by Katherine Oaks.*

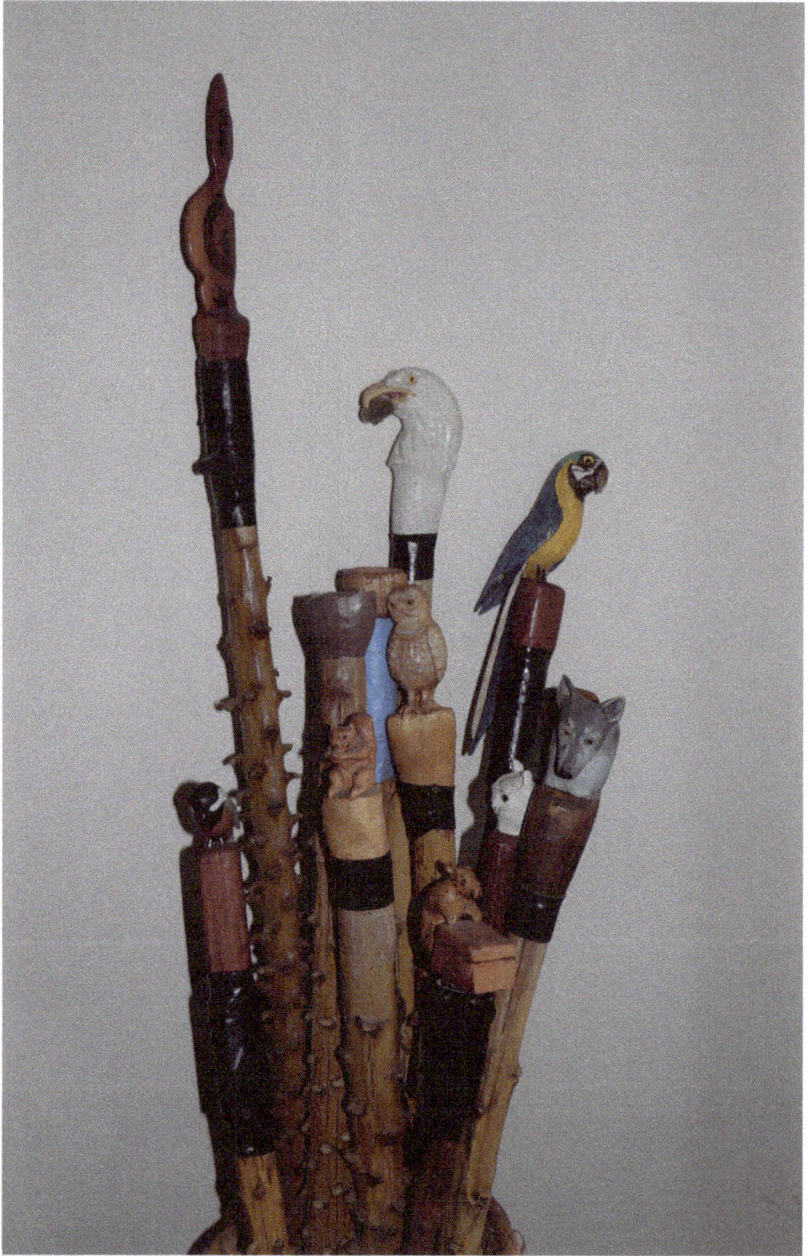

Fig. 8.12. Canes made by Barbara Hufford in 2001 from the flower stalks of coconut palms in Cape Coral, Florida. Each is topped with a carved figure meaningful to the recipients who attended a family reunion in celebration of Duane and Barbara's fiftieth wedding anniversary. *Photograph by Katherine Oaks.*

Figs 8.13, 8.14, and 8.15. Barbara's carved canes regularly drew passing pedestrians (and a few porch sitters) into conversation with her. *Photographs by Mary Hufford.*

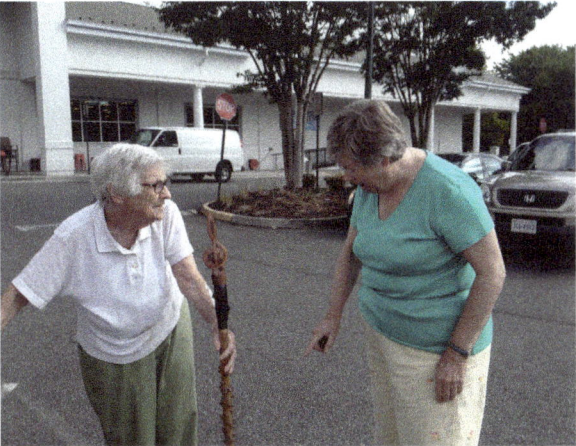

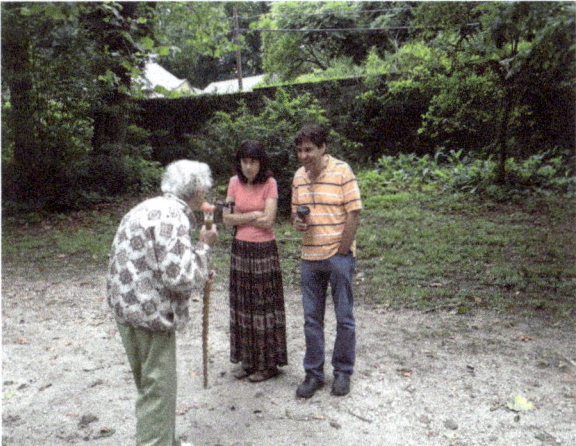

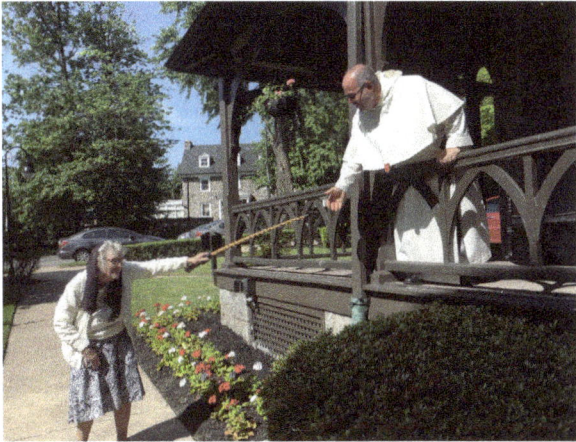

It is important to note that Barbara's carvings were not *memory* projects in the sense that she was reviewing her own life. Rather, in the last few decades of her life, her carvings bore witness to family life as it continued to unfold in far-flung places. The artistic celebration of life's "enduring and recurrent aspects" is especially important, I used to think, in families that have been scattered, a means of tempering modernity's fragmenting effects. But I see in my mother's carvings and in my fieldwork with communities in the Appalachian coalfields the work of elders in weaving larger ecological cycles together with biographical cycles into what Herbert Reid and Betsy Taylor (2010) call the Life Round.

Looking more closely at how elders weave times and cycles together takes us beyond the frame of individual human development, beyond the necessary work of life integration and the recovery of lost worlds through various kinds of life review. I have become interested in how elders through their communications engage a practice that I call "tending the flesh of sensibility," seeding collective sensibility by depositing memories in materials of the world, which we cannot help but harvest later in our own lives. David Abram (1996, 66) describes this flesh as a lining that gives rise to perceiver and perceived, subject and object, namer and named, as "interdependent aspects of its spontaneous activity."

Karl Marx called the senses a historical achievement. "The forming of the five senses," he wrote, "is a labor of the entire history of the world down to the present" (Marx 1844, 108). In recovering lost worlds from childhood through artistic representations and stories about them, elderly artists are in fact tending what is a historical sensibility. In the presence of such artifacts and their ingredient memories, we gain admission into what Merleau-Ponty (1968) calls Being—thereby coming to know ourselves to be part of a seeing, a hearing, a tasting, a sensing that is far older than our own and also far younger. It is a powerful invitation to inhabit what John O'Neill (1974), in *Making Sense Together*, calls time's body.

I'd like to illustrate this point with two examples, one from my mother and one from collaborators on Coal River, where I continue to do fieldwork. After my father's death, a year and half ago, my mother divided her time between our home in Bala Cynwyd, Pennsylvania, and my brother's home in the DC area. Bala Cynwyd is not far from where my mother spent most of her childhood, in Bryn Mawr, where she lived with her grandmother following her mother's death in 1936. My mother's father had grown up in Villanova. Both families occupied the same homes for three generations, before the properties were bought by Bryn Mawr College and Villanova University and the houses torn down. Because it jogged her memory, and she took pleasure in that, I regularly drove my mother along Old Gulph Road, which connects both family sites. She would often comment on things we passed, and I marveled at how the sights would trigger memories that no amount of inquiry could glean in the absence of those settings. One day, we drove across the four-lane bridge over the railroad tracks at

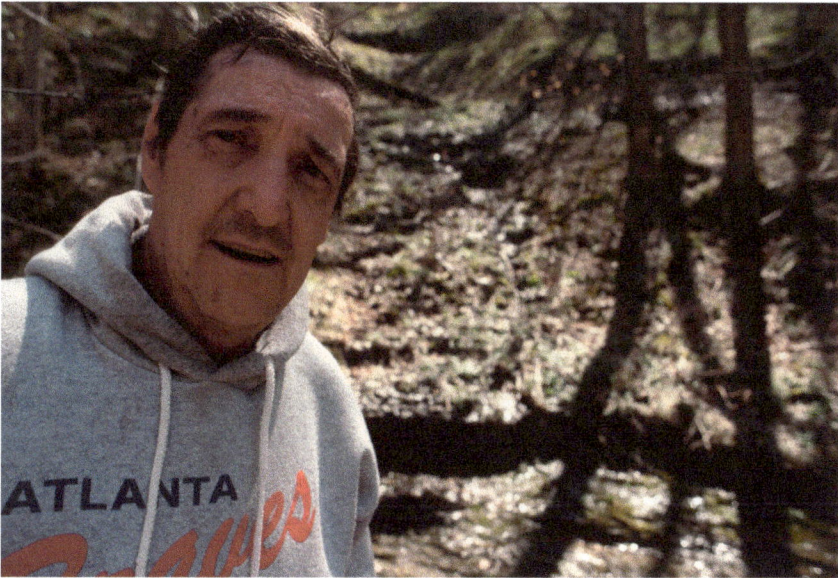

Fig. 8.16. David Bailey, near the head of Hazy Creek in April 1996. *Photograph by Lyntha Scott Eiler. Courtesy of the American Folklife Center.*

Villanova, and she exclaimed, "This bridge used to rattle when you drove over it. What happened to the rattle?" The construction of steel and concrete over which we drove that day had many decades earlier replaced the wooden bridge that told the Strongs of approaching vehicles. This explanation never satisfied Mom. "They should have kept the rattle!" she would say indignantly, each time we crossed over after that. I don't have to hold on to this memory received from my mother. It is lodged between me and that bridge, in recurring perceptual activity—in this case, seeing and hearing—that first deposits and then continually renews a flesh of sensibility. "The sensory landscape and its meaning-endowed objects," writes Nadia Seremetakis (1996, 7), "bear within them emotional and historical sedimentation that can provoke and ignite gestures, discourses, and acts." The silence of the bridge that lost its rattle haunts me now whenever I drive that way. It is a gift that keeps on giving, for, as Michel de Certeau (1984, 108) put it, "Haunted places are the only ones people can live in."

My other example comes from Coal River, a resource frontier, ground zero for mountaintop removal mining, where communities dominated by the coal industry have experienced acute forms of displacement while remaining in place (Hufford, 2009). Hanging on to history can be just as challenging for communities remaining in places that are disassembled and abandoned as it is for dispersed communities. David Bailey (fig. 8.16), a man now in his eighties,

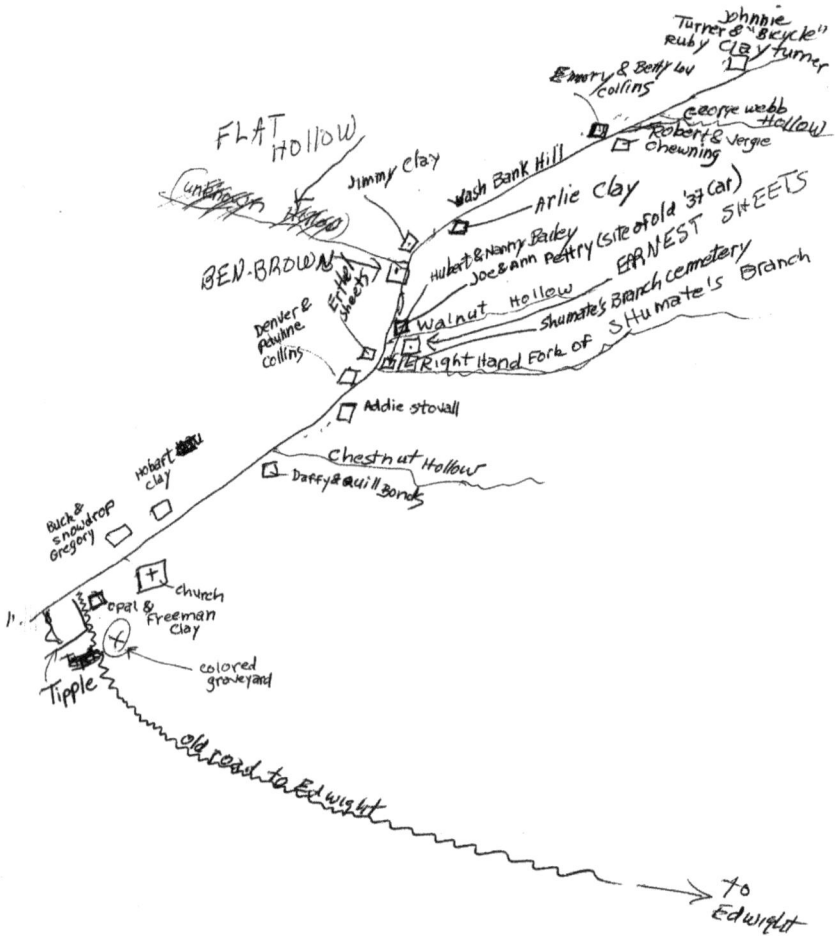

Shumate's Branch: Buildings, features, houses, etc.

Fig. 8.17. Map of the neighborhood of Shumate's Branch, brought to life in stories told by Dave Bailey. The agricultural community predating the Civil War was evacuated in the 1980s to make way for a coal waste impoundment. *Map created by Dave Bailey, Rick Bradford, and Charles Bradford.*

grew up in a hollow called Shumate's Branch. He is celebrated in his community as a gifted musician and storyteller. "You can just see everything he's telling about, the way he tells it," historian Rick Bradford of Edwight told me. Shumate's Branch was evacuated in the 1980s by Peabody Energy because the company needed a place in which to dispose of the waste water from the cleaning of coal. Dave Bailey, Rick Bradford, and others in the community memorialize the places

Figs 8.18, 8.19, and 8.20. Vehicles, re-created by Dave Bailey from cereal boxes, were familiar sights in Edwight and the surrounding hollows of Hazy Creek and Shumate's Branch. (left) Wilhoit's Cleaners and Driers and (right) the "Hazy Truck," a vehicle modified for the rugged terrain on Hazy Creek, a prime site for hunting, gathering, picnicking, fishing, and camping. *Photographs by Katherine Oaks.*

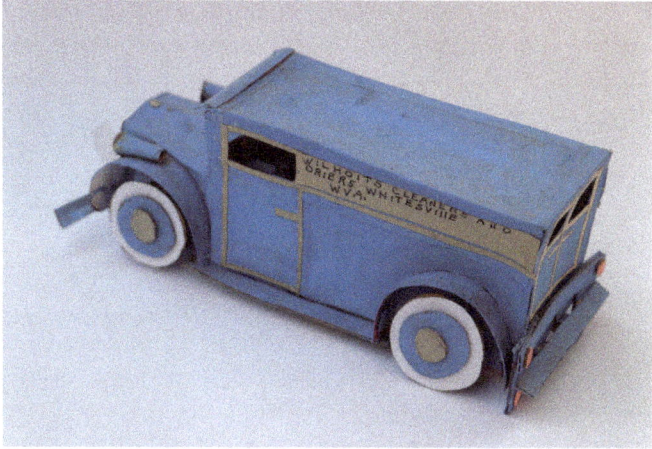

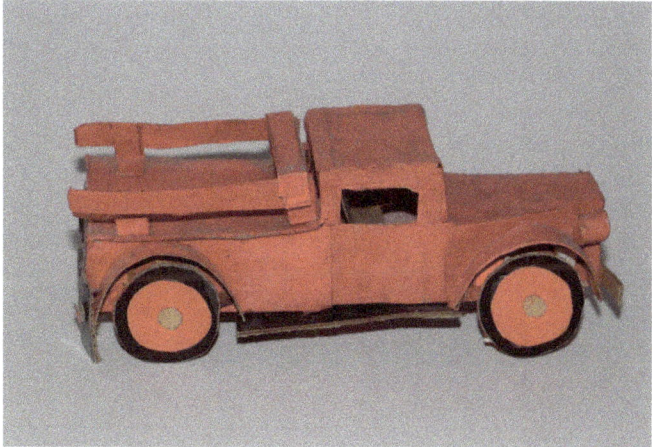

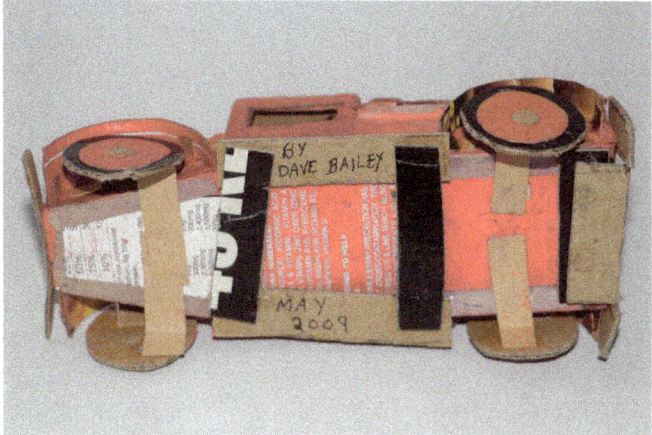

of Shumate's Branch, which had been a farming community for many generations, since before the Civil War. Bailey vividly recounts the stories of Shumate's
Branch at community gatherings, and Charles Bradford and his brother Rick
Bradford consulted with Dave Bailey to produce a map of the Shumate's Branch
neighborhood, brought to life through Dave's stories (fig. 8.17). Over the past few
years, Bailey has also been creating, out of cereal boxes, artifacts representing
the heyday of Shumate's Branch, Edwight, and Hazy Creek: the van driven by
the dry cleaner (fig. 8.18), and the Hazy truck (fig. 8.19), adapted for travel into
rugged places on Hazy Creek for camping and ginsenging—acoustically defined
places, back so far, as he put it, that you "couldn't hear the coal trucks." He paints
the artifacts, but the material history of each is preserved in the unpainted por-
tion (fig. 8.20), expressing a principle vital to the life round and to creative aging:
Everything can exceed itself to become something else. Everything can partake
of cycles of natality and mortality. Even trash—perhaps especially trash—can
become something more. Bailey's models prompt conversations and stories that
collectively redeposit and replenish a sensibility that in the dismantled places of
the coalfields languished decades ago.

In the Coal River Valley, a living intergenerational memory is deeply embedded in a seasonal round of gardening, hunting, and gathering on a forest commons (Hufford 1999). Names for hollows archive a flesh of sensibility—gener-
ations-ago things that people saw, heard, and practiced got talked about, and
the talk congealed into names from which historical sensory information can be
gleaned. I often ask people what they call the side hollows on their creeks. Several
times, in response, elders have rummaged through closets and drawers to locate
something on which they'd inscribe all those names: a flattened-out cigarette
carton or a scrap of drywall. These inscriptions are impelled by a sense of a world
vanishing, largely because, some people say, youth and elders are not talking to
each other as they used to. But there is another aspect to the story on Coal River,
which has for more than two decades now endured the devastating effects of
mountaintop removal mining. The retrieval of thin seams of coal by exploding
mountains has destroyed many of the upper elevation hollows and fragile wet-
land systems and associated histories of use commemorated in their names. Loss
of access to such places disrupts the multigenerational participation in shared
sensory experience. This disruption truncates the sense of participation in what
John O'Neill calls time's body. Defining time's body as "the time our senses need
to become human, to speak, and to think," O'Neill (1974, 37) addresses the need
for intergenerational collaboration in the renewal of human sensibility. Here, the
destruction of the land-base subtending that collaboration could be considered
an abrogation of what environmental ethicists call intergenerational rights (Wolf
2009). As Deborah Kapchan (2014, 22) notes, "In both narrative and non-narra-
tive forms . . . the right to sense and feel, the right to imagine, and the right to

identify are touchstones for intangible rights, sticky points of contact (see Tsing 2005) between the artificial separation of political, economic, cultural and social rights."

The function of nature as an active participant in the interweaving of multi-generational sensibilities bears on how we think about the interrelations of stages in the individual life cycle within larger generational cycles. Even though Edith Cobb's (1977) pioneering work on the ecology of imagination in childhood was published decades ago, we have not sufficiently appreciated its implications for the renewal of human sensibility as an intergenerational process. Cobb studied the middle stage of childhood, between the ages of six and twelve, to understand its bearing on the capacity for artistic work in adulthood. From her examination of dozens of biographies of well-known writers and artists, and her ethnographic observations of children at play, Cobb (1977, 16) concluded that world-making projects of children exhibit a "corresponding bioaesthetic striving" of child and nature "fundamental to the fulfillment of individual human biological develop-ment" (see also Reid and Taylor 2010, 134). Connecting the biocultural conti-nuities established in childhood projects with the developmental tasks of later life, Cobb (1977, 89) writes, "the child 'knows' or recognizes in these moments that he makes his own world and that his body is a unique instrument, where the powers of nature and human nature meet. These very moments are recalled autobiographically by the adult who seeks to renew and reinforce vision and so extend creative powers." Marx (1844, 108) had in a way anticipated Cobb's work in his insight that the human nature sense "comes to be by virtue of its object, by virtue of *humanized* nature."

Doing fieldwork over the *longue durée* in any place engages us in its cycles, and we may recognize that at play in those cycles are models for accessing and inhabiting time's body. When I met Wesley Scarbro, who volunteered on a citi-zen science forest monitoring project I worked with in the 1990s, he was in his twenties and newly married. He and his wife are now caring for grandchildren. As we sat on his porch overlooking the road and creek, I asked him about his butternut tree. Butternuts, also known as white walnuts, are not all that com-mon and are prized for their nutmeats as well as their timber. Wesley told me he's had offers for that tree, but he would never sell it. I asked if he collects the nuts. He said that he does and that people come from other places to gather his butternuts. An elderly woman came a few years ago, and he gave her permission to bring her grandchildren to gather butternuts. Now she does that every year, he said, and seeing her with her grandchildren prompts memories of gathering beechnuts and black walnuts on Buffalo Fork with his own grandmother when he was a child.

This, in a nutshell, if you will, is praxis exuding what Margaret Mead (1972) called "the human unit of time," which we explored in the last chapter of *The*

*Grand Generation* and which anticipates my present recourse to John O'Neill's notion of time's body. "Recurrent and enduring" activities that over the *longue durée* weave together the seasonal and generational cycles into a larger life round require intergenerational collaborations. I've become interested in how those collaborations, often structured into the kinds of forms that folklorists study, operate on sensibility, and how that sensibility can be a starting point for restoring and tending systems that are at once cultural and ecological, and in the complex collaborations of elders, children, and nature that curate time's body.

MARY HUFFORD is Director of Arts and Humanities for the Livelihoods Knowledge Exchange Network, a network for scholarly-community collaboration to build economic futures based on local assets, values, and vision. She is author of *Chaseworld: Foxhunting and Storytelling in New Jersey's Pine Barrens.*

## Works Cited

Abram, David. 1996. *The Spell of the Sensuous: Perception and Language in a More-Than-Human World.* New York: Vintage Books.

Byrd, Cynthia, curator. 2012. "Making Her Mark: A Showcase of Women Carvers." Ward Museum, Salisbury, MD, February 10–April 1.

Cobb, Edith. 1977. *The Ecology of Imagination in Childhood.* Dallas: Spring Publications.

De Certeau, Michel. 1984. *The Practice of Everyday Life.* Berkeley: University of California Press.

Hufford, Mary. 1999. "Seasonal Round of Activities on Coal River." American Folklife Center, Library of Congress. https://www.loc.gov/collections/folklife-and-landscape-in-southern-west-virginia/articles-and-essays/seasonal-round-of-activities-on-coal-river/.

Hufford, Mary. 2009. "Mountaintop Removal Mining." In *Encyclopedia of Environmental Ethics and Philosophy,* vol. 2, edited by J. Baird Callicott and Robert Frodeman, 63–68. Detroit: Gale Cengage.

Hufford, Mary, Marjorie Hunt, and Steven J. Zeitlin. 1987. *The Grand Generation: Memory, Mastery, Legacy.* Washington, DC: Smithsonian Institution.

Kapchan, Deborah, ed. 2014. *Cultural Heritage in Transit: Intangible Rights as Human Rights.* Philadelphia: University of Pennsylvania Press.

Kirshenblatt-Gimblett, Barbara. 1987. "Introduction." In *The Grand Generation: Memory, Mastery, Legacy,* edited by Mary Hufford, Marjorie Hunt, and Steven Zeitlin, 12–15. Washington, DC: Smithsonian Institution.

Marx, Karl. 1844. *Economic and Philosophic Manuscripts of 1844.* New York: Dover.

Mead, Margaret. 1972. *Blackberry Winter: My Earlier Years.* New York: William Morrow.

Mead, Margaret, and Rhoda Metraux. 1953. *The Study of Culture at a Distance.* Chicago: University of Chicago Press.

Merleau-Ponty, Merleau. 1968. *The Visible and the Invisible.* Evanston: Northwestern University Press.

O'Neill, John. 1974. *Making Sense Together: An Invitation to Wild Sociology.* New York: Harper.

Reid, Herbert, and Betsy Taylor. 2010. *Recovering the Commons: Democracy, Place, and Global Justice.* Urbana: University of Illinois Press.

Seremetakis, C. Nadia, ed. 1996. *The Senses Still: Perception and Memory as Material Culture in Modernity.* Chicago: University of Chicago Press.

Tsing, Anna. 2005. *Friction: An Ethnography of Global Connection.* Princeton: Princeton University Press.

Wolf, Clark. 2009. "Intergenerational Justice." In *Encyclopedia of Environmental Ethics and Philosophy*, vol. 1, edited by J. Baird Callicott and Robert Frodeman, 518–25. Detroit: Gale Cengage.

# PART II
# FOLKLIFE AND CREATIVE AGING PROGRAMS

# 9     Elderhood Arts

## Kathleen Mundell

Born in Motahkmikuk, Indian Township, Maine, Molly Neptune Parker is one of the most gifted basketmakers of the Passamaquoddy tribe. Now in her eighties, she has taught generations of Passamaquoddy tribal members including many of her children, grandchildren, and great-grandchildren. As both a keeper and a generator of Passamaquoddy culture, Molly Neptune Parker exemplifies what it means to be an elder. As she describes it: "Basket making is an art that I believe I was born to do, much as my ancestors have done for thousands of years. I honor that legacy and believe I have a responsibility to continue it" (fig. 9.1).

In many traditional cultures, the term *elder* confers a position of knowledge and authority, as elders take on their unique role of guiding and mentoring the next generation. But for those of us who have not benefitted from a culture that values or even recognizes the idea of elderhood, the process of growing older can be overwhelming. With its emphasis on physical and mental decline, the contemporary Western view of aging is often looked at as a problem: "Young is beautiful. Old is ugly. This attitude stems from a stereotyping deeply ingrained in our culture and in our economy. . . . The cruelest aspect of this cultural attitude is the elder's vulnerability to the stereotype. Some feel themselves to be unattractive, dull and quite often, unlovable, and this depressing outlook only aggravates the problem. One response is to avoid looking or acting your own age at all costs. Another attitude is to let go, renouncing even rewarding interests and pleasures as unseemly. The acceptance of the stereotype then actualizes the stereotype itself" (Erikson, Erickson, and Kivnick 1986, 301).

In contrast is the recognition of elderhood as a distinct and significant phase of life—one that affords older adults new opportunities to take on new roles as teachers, grandparents, mentors, and advocates for the future: "By relegating this

*The Expressive Lives of Elders* (2018): 175–185, DOI: 10.2979/expressivelivesofelders.0.0.10

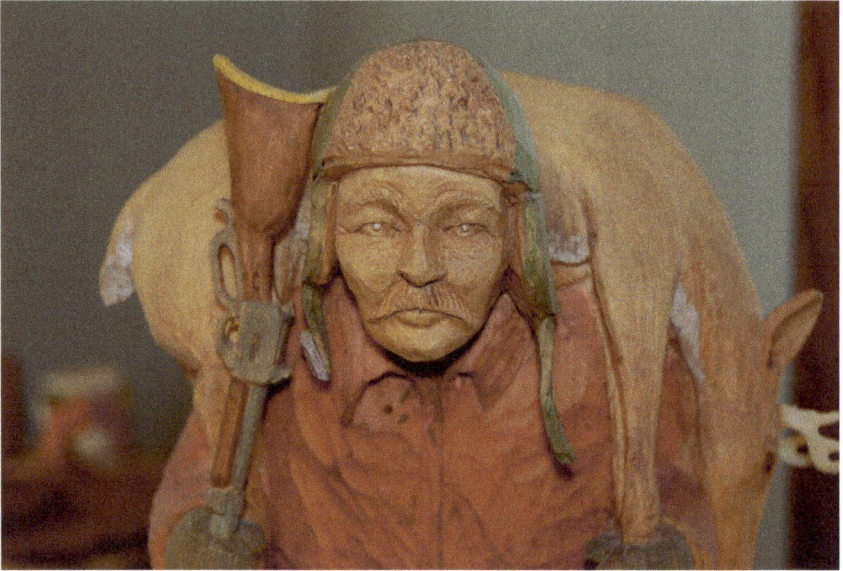

Fig. 9.1. Acadian Hunter by Tom Cote. *Photograph by Peter Dembski.*

growing segment of the population to the onlooker bleachers of our society, we have classified them as unproductive, inadequate, and inferior. . . . Taking care of them in innumerable ways is being responsible. Entertaining them with bingo games and concerts is, however, patronizing. Surely, the search for some way of including what they can still contribute to the social order in a way befitting their capacities is appropriate and in order" (Erikson, Erikson, and Kivnick 1986, 301).

Elderhood is also a phase of life in which older adults get a chance to tap into their life experiences and creatively tell their stories. As folklorists Mary Hufford, Marjorie Hunt, and Steve Zeitlin (1987, 41) suggest, "No matter how it comes about, telling one's story seems an essential part of being an elder, and culture provides an array of expressive forms for putting one's story forth."

The process of looking inward is a natural part of growing older. As psychoanalyst Erik Erikson (1982, 65) suggests, exploring a deeper sense of self is part of this stage of life, what he refers to as the point of integrity in which "we have come to the point of being able to understand our place in the world and the life we have lived in it." This life chapter, explains Erikson (1950, 268) is "where one can look back at life and accept it as it has come to be." Such acceptance is part of becoming an elder, freeing us to serve others and giving back all that our own life experience has given us.

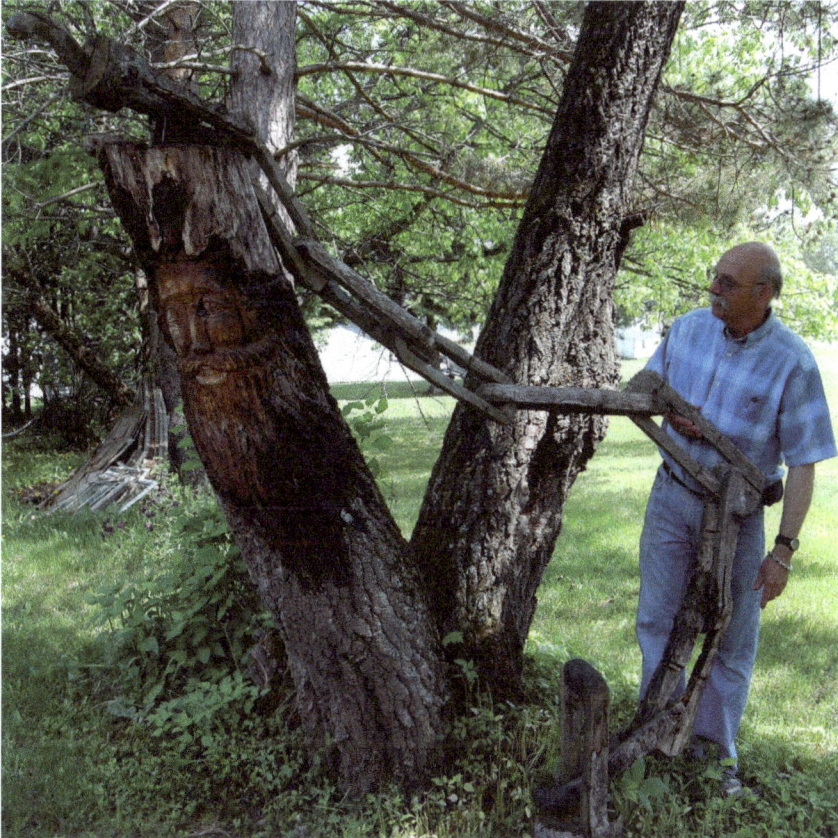

Fig. 9.2. Woodcarver Tom Cote with carved wooden chain. *Photograph by Peter Dembski.*

The journey of self-exploration often expresses itself in creative ways. Creativity comes from the Latin *creatus*, which means "to have grown." Central to this idea is the recognition of how creativity affects the aging brain. More than two decades ago, Gene Cohen, renowned geriatric psychiatrist and director of the Center for Aging, Health & Humanities at George Washington University, suggested that creativity was like "chocolate" for the brain. Cohen's landmark research pointed to the positive impact of creativity on older adults' physical, mental, and emotional health. He coined the term *creative aging* to describe how creativity, in all its multifaceted forms, can not only help sharpen cognitive skills but also further the aging brain's ability to grow, change, and form new connections (Cohen 2006, 7–15).

Out of the Cohen's research and the continued work of the National Center for Creative Aging, the creative aging field has grown steadily with new and innovative programs developed to enhance older adults' ability to advance their artistic abilities. Still, the definitions of what is "creativity" with its emphasis on "fine art" and its push toward professional teaching artists delivering art instruction to older adults remains narrowly defined. Such an approach overshadows the potential for older adults to be inspired by their own lives and cultural traditions, as folklorist Alan Jabbour (1982, 24) explains: "Folk arts mean fundamentally drawing out special forms of expression, people already possess, not laying on arts, forms or programs they lack."

As the arts and aging field moves forward, recognizing and nurturing these special forms of expressive culture is crucial in helping older adults sustain meaning and renewed purpose. Traditional arts such as basket making, quilting, woodcarving, cooking, weaving, gardening, canning, storytelling, singing, music, and dancing hold great meaning in the lives of older adults and their communities. Reflecting the values and practices of a shared culture based on geography, language, religion, occupation, ethnic heritage, tribal affiliation, or family background, these expressions are learned in an informal way, usually through observation and example, and are individually crafted, traditionally learned, and community shared. As symbols of family heritage, cultural identity, and artistic inheritance, such expressions have much meaning for those who continue to practice them (fig. 9.2).

As a nonprofit working with traditional artists and communities on honoring and sustaining their cultural traditions, Cultural Resources often works with elders. Our Elderhood Arts program honors the idea of elders as keepers of their culture as well as celebrates their important role in acting as connecting points for family and community culture. Through a range of programs, Elderhood Arts offers older adults and healthcare professionals an opportunity to discover and recognize the significant role cultural traditions can play in the lives of older adults.

In designing the Elderhood Arts program, we turned to many resources in the field of creativity and aging including the work of Gene Cohen, Susan Perlstein, and folklorists Barbara Kirshenblatt-Gimblett, Mary Hufford, Marjorie Hunt, Steven Zeitlin, Jon Kay, and Troyd Geist. Particularly useful was the work of Erik Erikson and his ideas about human development through the life cycle. In describing the seventh phase in the life cycle, Erikson developed the concept of generativity. Defining *generativity* as "a concern for establishing and guiding the next generation," an indicator of an elderhood, he suggested, is the need and ability to look beyond yourself and care for others (Erikson 1982, 107).

In exploring the relationship between creativity, the generative process, and healthy aging, Cultural Resources collaborated on the development of a training program called Living Arts/Living Well Studio. Our partner was the University of New England Geriatric Education Center, an organization that offers professional development seminars for healthcare professionals in hospitals and assisted living centers. The goal was to show healthcare providers how overall well-being improves when caregivers take a person-centered approach, getting to know their patients as whole human beings with unique abilities and experiences.

The series took place at various hospitals and assisted living centers throughout Maine from 2012 to 2016 and featured master traditional artists from the Maine Arts Commission's Traditional Arts Apprenticeship Program as role models of elderhood. With the support of the National Endowment for the Arts, Maine's Traditional Arts Apprenticeship Program works with traditional artists and their communities in sustaining their cultural heritage by providing opportunities for master traditional artists to pass on their skills to an apprentice of their choice. The program acts as a kind of cultural aquifer, encouraging elder master artists to teach valuable skills and cultural knowledge to younger generations.

More than just transferring artistic skills, apprenticeships also establish important personal and cultural relationships. The intricate and overlapping relationships of elder and apprentice, grandparent and grandchild, friend and neighbor, are constantly at play as techniques, creative ideas, and cultural knowledge are exchanged. Now sixty years old, Theresa Secord was once an apprentice to Penobscot basketmaker and elder Madeline Tomer Shay. Secord has gone on to be a master in her own right and is the founding director of Maine Indian Basketmakers Alliance, an intertribal organization dedicated to the preservation of the sweet grass and brown ash basketry tradition. Secord describes the impact of the apprenticeship program as "a catalyst for many of us who are continuing the work. As an apprentice to Madeline Tomer Shay in 1990, I first became aware that after hundreds, perhaps thousands of years, our basket-making traditions were slipping away. At that time, I was one of only a dozen Maine Indians younger than the age of fifty who were practicing the tradition. Then in 1993, Madeline Shay, my teacher died. It was then that I began my own teaching in the apprenticeship program, determined not to watch this tradition die."

The traditional master artists featured in the Living Art/Living Well Studio workshops embody the values of elderhood. Growing up in a basket-making family, Molly Neptune Parker likes to remember how everyone worked together on ash baskets: "Some would work on fancy baskets and some would make work baskets, like the scale baskets made to hold fish scales from the sardine factory." Making and selling ash and sweet grass baskets has always been a tradition among the Wabanaki (Passamaquoddy, Penobscot, Micmac, and Maliseet) of Maine (fig. 9.3).

In sharing her life story with healthcare professionals, Parker has created what gerontologists' term a generativity script: "Basket making to me is about

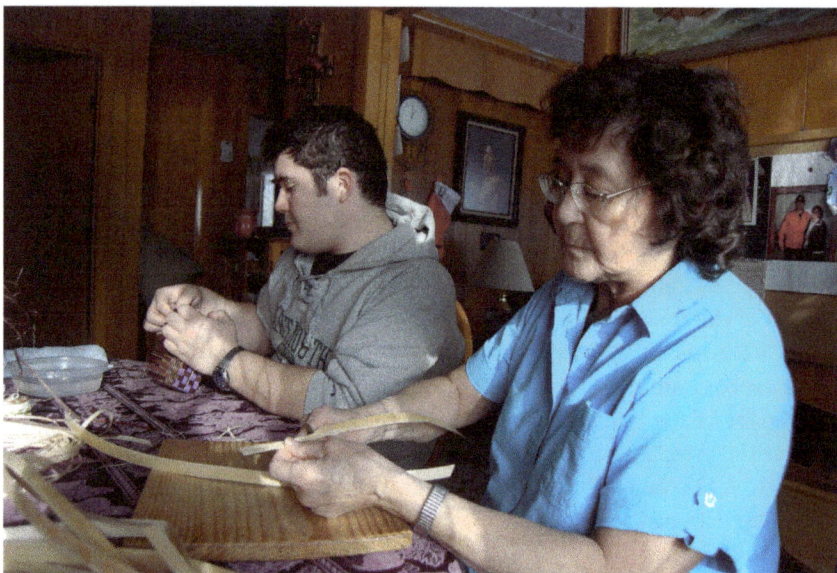

Fig. 9.3. Molly Neptune Parker with grandson Geo Neptune. *Photograph by Peter Dembski.*

our respect for using the bounty of nature and the talent of generations in making something of value, beauty, and function. The art of Passamaquoddy basket making has been woven throughout all aspects of my life. I have used it to teach myself, my children, my grandchildren, and others about Passamaquoddy traditions, history, values, and language." The generativity script is "an inner narration of the adult's own awareness of where efforts to be generative fit into his or her own personal history, into contemporary society and the social world he or she inhabits, and in some extraordinary cases, into society's own encompassing history" (McAdams and de St. Aubin 1992, 1006).

Because of Parker's lifelong commitment to her culture, a younger generation will continue to work with traditional materials, methods, and styles. Created within a circle of history, the generative script helps strengthen the role of the elder while also transforming older forms of art into a living contemporary community tradition. As her grandson and apprentice Geo Neptune explains, "I know when I'm older and my grandmother is no longer around to make baskets, I'll be making my style, but I will also be making more traditional baskets. I'll be making baskets with her in mind" (fig. 9.4).

Another artist featured in Living Arts/Living Well is master woodcarver Tom Cote. Cote comes from a long line of talented woodcarvers, stretching as

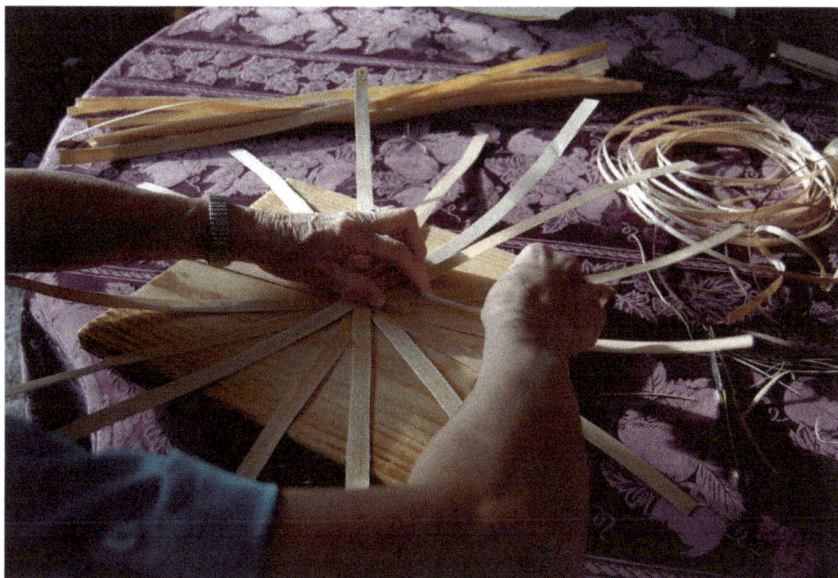

Fig. 9.4. Passamaquoddy basketmaker Molly Neptune Parker weaving a basket. *Photograph by Peter Dembski.*

far back as his great-great-grandfather Jean Baptiste Cote of Quebec, a carver of church altars. In his studio in Limestone, Maine, Tom says carving continues to remind him of growing up in Maine's St. John Valley. Settled in 1785, the St. John Valley is home to a vibrant French-speaking population, tracing its roots to Acadia and Quebec. Learning the basics of carving from his mother and grandfather at age twelve, Tom Cote, now in his late seventies, eventually went on to apprentice with a cousin and woodcarver in Saint-John-Port-Joli, Quebec.

Cote continues to teach a new generation of woodcarvers, including his granddaughter, Ellyabeth Bencivenga: "I want to teach my apprentices that carvers have a tradition of dealing with the shaping of dull, common, and ordinary things into objects of interest and value, using local raw materials to enrich the lives of family and friends. This is an important part of the Acadian tradition. Carvers made items that were useful for everyday living from spoons to cookie boards to molding used in homes. And they made items that were just inspirational, like the carved altars in the local churches and the sculptures that depicted local saints and religious figures" (fig. 9.5).

Malcolm Knowles suggests that older adults are more self-directed than their younger counterparts and are drawn to challenges that call for problem

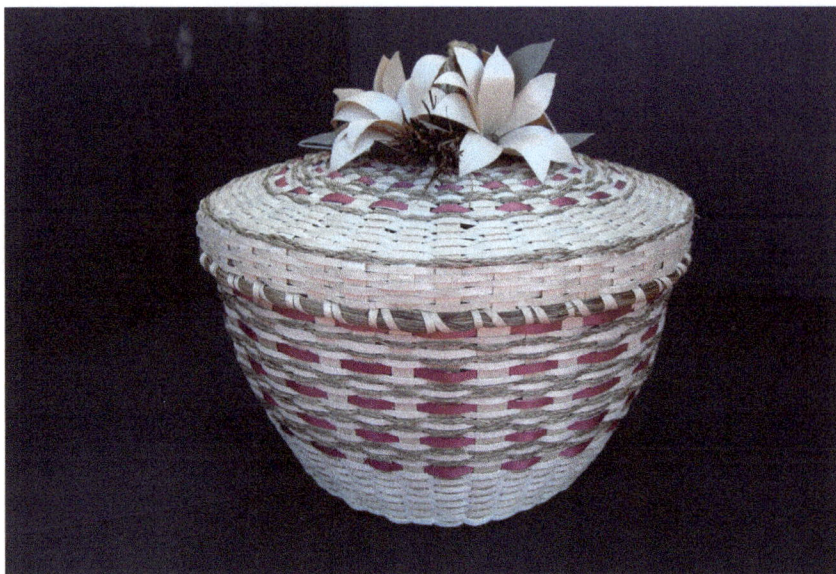

Fig. 9.5. Ash and sweet grass basket by Molly Neptune Parker. *Photograph by Peter Dembski.*

solving and hands-on engagement—a learning style he terms andragogy. Elders, he found, learn best in collaborative, process-oriented settings, as opposed to more traditional, didactic approaches centered on merely conveying content. They are especially motivated by topics and activities that are relevant to their life experiences (Knowles 1984, 5).

Evident in Cote's beautifully carved murals, depicting such Acadian and regional traditions as deer hunting, sawing wood for firewood, potato harvesting, and maple syruping, is his deep connection to his place: "Inspiration for my work comes from history and places, things and people I have seen throughout my life. Research and the details of the item or person are very important to create the details and to make sure it is historically correct is the aspect of my work and something to which I find I am very sensitive. Whenever I create a piece, I am most pleased when someone understands the personal connection behind my work" (fig. 9.6).

For many, the generative process begins with the past, reviewing life experiences in order to share it with others. This unfolding process, by which we take stock of ourselves and our lives, is called life review. Developed by gerontologist Robert Butler (1963), life review is the process of self-reflection and reevaluation of life events. Butler based the idea of life review on Erik Erikson's ideas about

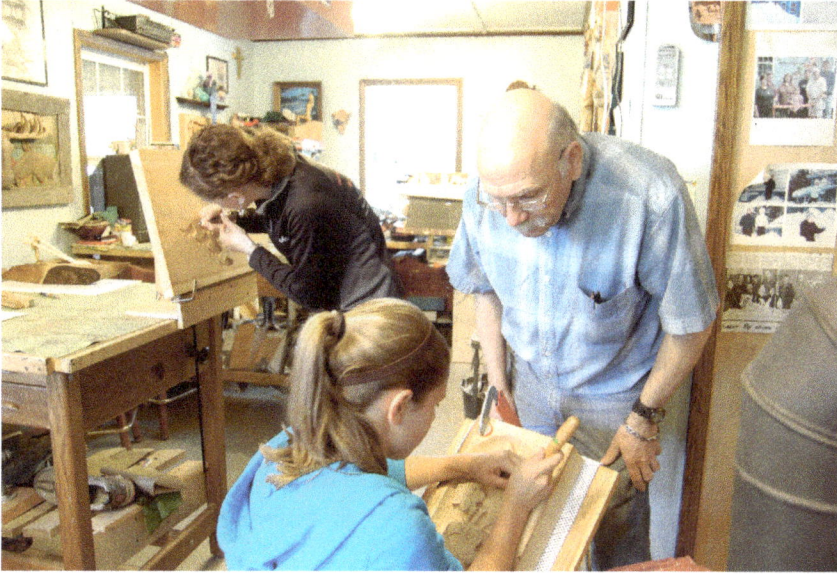

Fig. 9.6. Woodcarver Tom Cote teaching apprentices. *Photograph by Peter Dembski.*

integration and the developmental stages of the life cycle. In doing so, he created a new way for people to think about their past. Butler's work also proved to be influential in changing the prevailing negative attitude toward the role of reminiscence in the aging process. Once considered a sign of cognitive decline, remembering plays an important role in healthy aging.

The life review process, offers people a chance to explore, organize, and curate narratives about specific chapters of their lives. This imaginative recycling of events often helps make sense of and even reconcile experiences. As Carl Jung (1971, 22) explains, "Life review involves a critical examination of one's life leading toward reconciliation between the sweet and the sour in life. It is a process for removing regret and anger from one's worldview."

Primarily used in therapeutic settings, life review techniques can also be used as the raw material for creative expressions. Through a series of workshops geared toward older adults, Cultural Resources recently developed Place Stamp Here, a program that explores the process of life review through interviewing techniques, memory maps, journal writing, poetry, and drawing. These exercises are used to not only organize and revaluate experiences but also to stir the pot for creative ways to share these experiences. The end result is a life story portfolio. Keeping in mind who is the audience for this material is part of creating the portfolio. Early on, participants are encouraged to pick a person who will be a recipient of the finished portfolio and write a letter about Place Stamp Here workshop to see if they are interested in participating.

Each week, such topics as family background, work, childhood, young adulthood, adulthood, and elderhood are explored. For each life chapter, participants are encouraged to create a corresponding visual image, a poem, a song, or a piece of writing. These exercises help people to start thinking about life experiences in a metaphorical way. They often reframe events as well as transform a new perspective for both the creator and the intended audience.

In organizing and sharing these experiences, we first ask people to begin by thinking about what parts of their lives do they feel a need to express. Early on, we ask a series of questions: Out of the thousands of events in your lifetime, select five that significantly shaped the direction of your life, and then, how do you organize these events in your mind? Does it break down into eras? Or where you lived at different times? What were some of the turning points of your life?

This process is not a literal, linear march through time but an occasion for metaphorical thinking and what Albert Einstein (Hadamard 1945, 142–43) called combinatory play or the "act of opening up one mental channel by dabbling in another." It takes complementary creative activities such as writing and drawing and generates new associations about past memories. For example, in reviewing stories about occupational experiences, participants are asked to focus on an event or a series of events that speaks to their work lives. This can be a poem, a proverb, a short description, or even a list of all the jobs that can be remembered. These reflections are then combined with drawing of hands.

Such creative work calls for looking at life differently, reframing chapters to transform new meaning and points of view. Although Elderhood Arts is off to a good start, there remains much to be done. An emphasis on creativity—on helping people reach within themselves to find meaning and connection—will remain central as we continue to bring older adults together to rediscover and strengthen their personal worth and social capital.

KATHLEEN MUNDELL is Director of the Elderhood Arts Program at Cultural Resources in Rockport, Maine. She is author of *North by Northeast: Wabanaki, Haudenosaunee and Tuscarora Traditional Arts.*

## Works Cited

Butler, Robert N. 1963. "The Life Review: An Interpretation of Reminiscence in the Aged." *Psychiatry* 26 (1): 65–67.

Cohen, Gene D. 2006. Research on Creativity and Aging: The Positive Impact of the Arts on Health and Illness. *Generations* 30 (1): 7–15

Erikson, E. H. 1963. *Childhood and Society.* New York: Norton.

Erikson, E. H. 1982. *The Life Cycle Completed.* Norton: New York

Erikson, E. H., J. Erikson, and H. Kivnick. 1986. *Vital Involvement in Old Age.* New York: Norton.

Hadamard, Jacques. 1945. *An Essay on the Psychology of Invention in the Mathematical Field.* Princeton, NJ: Princeton University Press.

Hufford, Mary, Marjorie Hunt, and Steven Zeitlin. 1987. *The Grand Generation: Memory, Mastery, Legacy.* Washington, DC: Smithsonian Institution.

Jabbour, Alan. 1982. "Some Thoughts from a Folk Cultural Perspective." In *Perspectives on Aging*, edited by Priscilla W. Johnston, 139–49. Cambridge, MA: Ballinger.

Jung, C. G. 1971. *The Portable Jung*, ed. J. Campbell. New York: Viking.

Knowles, Malcolm S. 1984. *The Adult Learner: A Neglected Species.* Houston: Gulf.

McAdams, Dan P., and Ed de St. Aubin. 1992. "A Theory of Generativity and Its Assessment through Self-Report, Behavioral Acts, and Narrative Themes in Autobiography." *Journal of Personality and Social Psychology* 62 (6): 1003–15.

# 10   Dancing Chairs and Mythic Trees

## *The Power of Folk Arts in Creative Aging, Health, and Wellness*

### Troyd Geist

OUR ELDERS ARE the most productive facilitators and largest repositories of folklore, folk art, and folk material culture (fig. 10.1). They also are among the greatest beneficiaries of that body of knowledge, practice, and way of life. And, ironically, they may be the ones most in need of the positive impact folk culture engenders in relation to health and wellness.

In the mid-1990s, as the folklorist with the North Dakota Council on the Arts (NDCA) directing its Folk and Traditional Arts Program, I began developing projects and programs with an eye toward the intersection of folk art, health, and well-being. Among those efforts, for example, is the creation of an exhibit of Ojibwa birch bark pictographic scrolls. This rare tradition involves the telling of ancient narratives in an elaborate series of pictographs. Traditional stories are still with us because they address issues that remain a part of the human condition. Each "written" scroll depicts a story that includes themes such as unrequited love, self-esteem, and violence. Unfortunately, these are issues with which today's children continue to grapple just as did past generations. Translations of the stories along with activity plans were developed and used as a counseling tool in schools. The exhibit toured extensively and clearly illustrated the power and accessibility of folk material culture as a tool to impact well-being.

Another example involves the utilization of storytelling as a counseling mechanism for the biological and adoptive families and their children impacted by fetal alcohol syndrome. Or the use of folk art and folklore in traditional gardening to address challenges associated with nutrition, diabetes, and cultural re-

*The Expressive Lives of Elders* (2018): 186–204, DOI: 10.2979/expressivelivesofelders.0.0.11

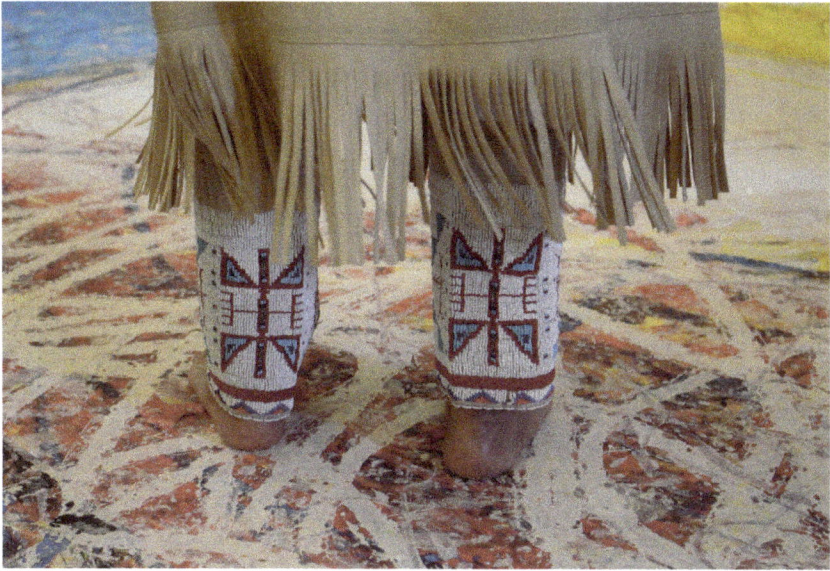

Fig. 10.1. Mary Louise Defender Wilson leads elders in creating a painting through traditional Dakota Sioux dance. *Courtesy of North Dakota Council on the Arts.*

tention. Some efforts like the traditional gardening project have been taken over and continued by the community in some form or another over the years since. While most of these projects were one-time activities, I also considered ways in which additional impact could be created from existing, ongoing programs.

Specifically with regard to the health and wellness of elders, the agency's targeted actions began in 1998–1999 as a spin-off from the public presentation requirement of the NDCA's long-standing Folk and Traditional Arts Apprenticeship Program. This program fosters the perpetuation and growth of folk arts by supporting master artists who teach apprentices one-on-one and face-to-face. Over a two-year period, I worked to schedule performances and presentations by apprenticeship program participants in nearly every eldercare facility in the state. Powerful anecdotes surfaced as to the association of those interactions with the elders' well-being. For example, a disassociated, immobile woman in a wheelchair tapping her finger to the songs and music of folk musicians. Or a man who, after many years, was able to dance again with his Alzheimer's disease–stricken wife. In many cases, such occasions left as profound impressions on the eldercare staff and artists as on the elders themselves.

In 1999, Lila Hauge-Stoffel and Mary O-Reilly Seim received a small apprenticeship grant to teach and learn traditional textile arts and the use of natural dyes. Lila first learned informally as a child to weave and color fiber while darning socks and tending the garden with her grandmother. Later, as an adult, she became a professor of art with an interest in therapeutic arts. At the time of the grant award, Mary worked as an activities director for an eldercare facility in Fargo, North Dakota. While the reported stories from their public presentation and that of other apprenticeship program folk artists were compelling, Lila, Mary, and I wondered if such interaction could be quantified regarding the health and wellness of elders.

So, from 2001 to 2003, with grant support from the National Endowment for the Arts, we developed and coordinated a small-sample, pilot study in the care facility where Mary worked. We sought to measure the effects of intensive arts and artist interaction on what William Thomas (1999, 11) identified as the Three Plagues—loneliness, boredom, and helplessness—which is detrimental to the health and wellness of elders in care facilities. Artist expressions utilized included quilting, storytelling, natural dyes, Swedish Dala painting, and more. Thirty-five sessions were held with residents whose average age was eighty-six. A self-evaluation tool of fifteen questions for each of the three "plagues" was utilized prior to the project's beginning, after each session, and upon conclusion of the project. At the end of two years, these arts interventions resulted in clearly positive improvement in loneliness, boredom, and, to a lesser extent, helplessness. The positive developmental change on a scale of 1 to 100 for various assessment questions moved as much as 36.4 points for the better. Again, powerful testimonies were noted.

For instance, Dala painting is a vibrant folk art tradition used to commemorate important family, community, and historical events in a colorful, framed series of decorative images. Pieper Bloomquist, a nurse and Dala painter, visited with a group of elders, some with memory issues. They discussed and shared experiences from their past, those that occurred when they were children or young adults. Frequently, with age-onset dementia it is the short-term memory of elders that is negatively affected first while long-term memory, ironically, is more enduring. Those memories that are held more dear and are older often involve such things as weddings, holidays with parents and siblings, special foods, and other things learned and experienced as we grow up—our folk culture.

One man in that group of elders sometimes would leave his room and become confused, lost, and upset. The care facility staff would have to find, comfort, and return him to his room. Pieper helped that man create a colorful, highly visible Dala painting based on a memory he shared in her painting workshop. The artwork of each participating elder was hung outside the door of their respective rooms. This man, still sometimes disoriented, often would recognize his painting, his memory from long ago, displayed outside his door. The art became a touchstone that allowed him to recognize and find his "home."

What did this do? It returned some independence, freedom, and sense of dignity to this man. It helped prevent stress hormones from raging throughout his body. It saved staff time dedicated to calming him and returning him to his room. It lessened the likelihood of needing expensive medications for sedation resulting in both health and financial benefits. Traditional art is powerful with regard to wellness, especially when it is thoughtfully, creatively, and practically engaged.

Based on these efforts and informed by many medical studies regarding the connection between art, aging, and wellness, I initiated the NDCA's statewide Art for Life Program. This program seeks to improve the emotional and physical health of elders in care facilities by fostering ongoing art and artist interaction through partnerships that include in each community a local arts agency, eldercare facility, folk and contemporary artists, and school. To augment the program for existing partners and to expand the concept to other communities, a toolkit with activity plans was developed over the course of five years.

Working with folklorists, academics, physicians, nurses, speech therapists, and folk and contemporary artists, dozens of plans, all based and contextualized with folklore and accompanied by synopses of sample medical studies, were developed with the support of the Bush Foundation. Distributed to 1,200 local arts agencies, eldercare facilities, and other organizations regionally and nationally in fall 2017, these plans are intended to guide communities in creative work with elders with an eye toward health and wellness.

When working with material folk art, aging, and wellness, several points are important to consider: (1) the creative process as well as the final object itself are crucial to impact; (2) activating the five senses, sometimes by integrating nonmaterial folk arts, folklore, or traditions such as food, music, or dance, can help enliven the elder in the process and toward the completion of the material art; and (3) interaction between elders in care facilities must be fostered. The creation of material folk art with these elements in mind can help trigger the positive health impacts related to the "sense of control mechanism," psychoneuroimmunology (PNI), nostalgia, life review, and the Proust phenomenon.

To illustrate, let us discuss two examples of projects guided by Art for Life Program activity plans. One employs nonmaterial folk arts—traditional dance—in the creation of monumental, contemporary paintings. The other engages conversations and folk traditions in the creation of a seven-foot-tall papercutting.

The first, Yes, I Am Free: The Inspiration of Dance and Paint, took place in four North Dakota communities—Jamestown, Ellendale, Enderlin, and Wahpeton—within our Art for Life Program network in 2015. It was designed by Jeff Nachtigall and me. Jeff is an internationally recognized artist from the Canadian province of Saskatchewan whose practice includes residencies with medical and care facilities. We partnered with a local arts agency and an eldercare facility in each community and worked with traditional artists Maureen McDonald-Hins (Irish dance), Margaret Sam (Bharatanatyam dance), James "Cubby" LaRocque (Michif fiddle music and jigging), and Mary Louise Defender Wilson (Dakota

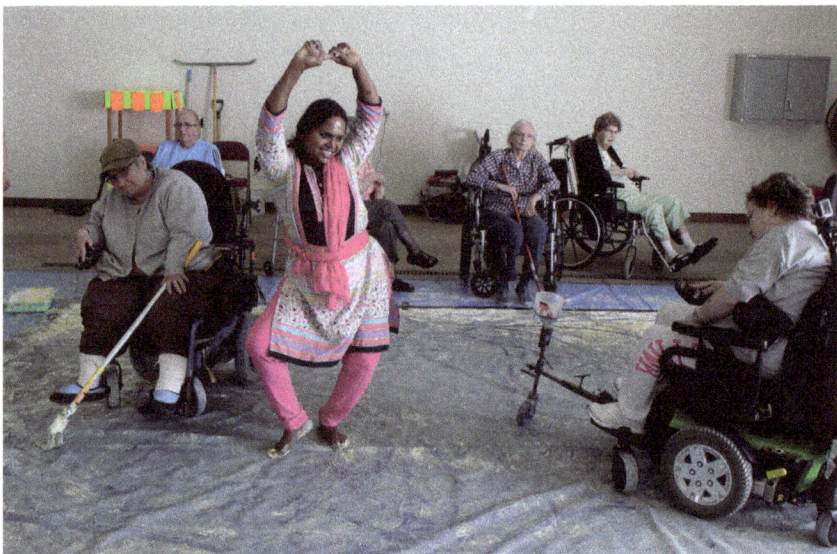

Fig. 10.2. Margaret Sam, East Indian Bharatanatyam dancer, with care facility residents, Jamestown, North Dakota. One resident uses the MPD while another uses an improvised mark-making device. *Courtesy of North Dakota Council on the Arts.*

dance). Also, let us not forget the heart of the creative process, the elders in the care facilities. While simple in concept, the project was creative and complex in planning and execution.

Imagine a twelve-by-fifteen-foot canvas on the floor. With rags tied to the bottom of strollers or walkers, to the ends of canes or broom handles, and with feet all dipped in paint, as music plays, the elders are guided in movement by the folk dancers. As they participate and on the canvas, they leave behind the rhythmic pattern of the dance. For people with more challenging mobility issues, the Mobile Painting Device (MPD) was utilized (fig. 10.2). Invented by Jeff, the MPD is basically a fifth-wheel attached to a wheelchair that acts as a giant paintbrush allowing the person to apply broad calligraphic brushstrokes as they "dance" across the canvas. The first day is loose and free in structure allowing the elders to release inhibitions, have fun, and better understand the process necessary for the following day (fig. 10.3).

On the second day, after the "base" of paint has dried, the same process as before is followed. However, it is more structured and controlled with Jeff and the traditional dancers collaborating more thoughtfully with regard to patterning or design, placement of paint, and which paints to use and when. This is required to avoid the muddling of colors and to enhance their blending into a pleasing effect.

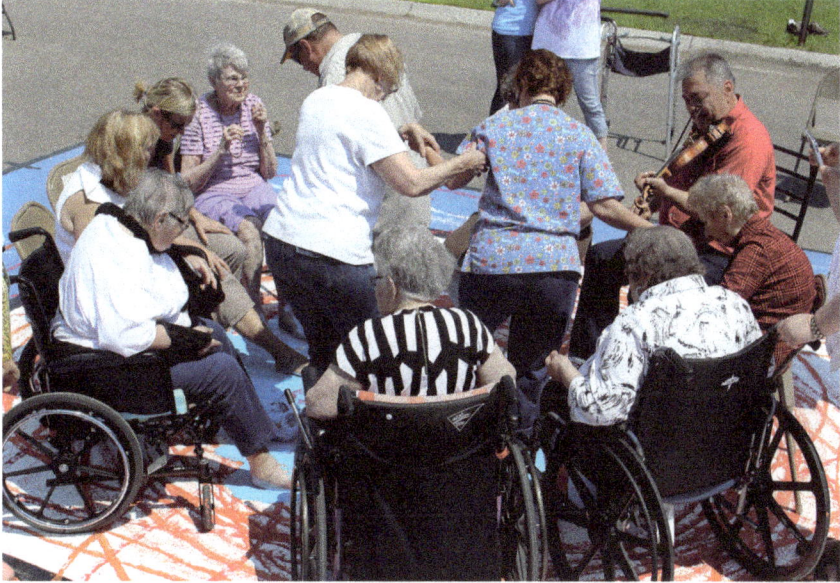

Fig. 10.3. James "Cubby" LaRocque performs Michif fiddle music while elders seated in their chairs jig, moving paint around the canvas with their feet, Wahpeton, North Dakota. *Courtesy of North Dakota Council on the Arts.*

The colors of acrylic paint were chosen based on their cultural association with the specific traditional dance performed. For example, green for Irish or the four colors of the medicine wheel for the Dakota. This was done to visually contextualize the contemporary paintings within the folk culture featured and to help ensure each of the four paintings would be unique.

The traditionalists also gave careful thought to the cultural meaning of the dance in which they guided the elders. For example, when selecting traditional dances and music, Mary Louise chose those that are, within the Dakota culture, associated with ceremonies for health and healing. The process of painting with each step, furthermore, was designed to visually create a medicine wheel, a powerful traditional symbol of interconnectedness and health (fig. 10.4).

One of the Irish folk dances Maureen led was based on the concept of two groups of strangers, suspicious of one another, meeting. She provided actual shillelaghs, the famed Irish fighting stick and cane, to be used by the elders in the dance. Explaining the cultural significance and use of these objects, Maureen directed the movement as elders approached one another from the corners and edges of the canvas, meeting in the middle, circling one another, and interweaving. With rags taped to the ends of the sticks dipped in paint, the elders were

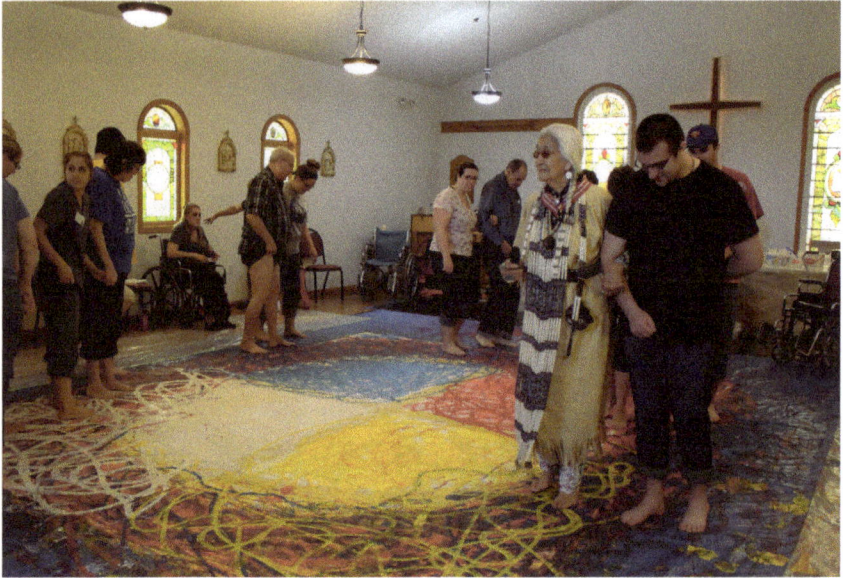

Fig. 10.4. Mary Louise Defender Wilson, Dakota Sioux traditionalist, with young people assisting elders in the creation of a medicine wheel painting, Ellendale, North Dakota. *Courtesy of North Dakota Council on the Arts.*

instructed to use the canes, tapping them against the canvas on the floor as they danced (fig. 10.5). Gently, at first, in their approach. Then harder and more vigorously as they met in the middle. Here, Maureen instructed the elders to hit the sticks harder and faster on the canvas to release their frustrations, worries, and fears. Once tired, Maureen explained that at this point, the strangers realize they have nothing to fear from one another and that they can be friends. Whereupon the elders were asked to again tap the shillelaghs gently as they were guided in their return to the outer edges of the canvas.

Ponder for a moment if someone said, "You are going to create a wall-sized contemporary painting. And you're going to do it with your feet, walkers, and canes." What would you think? For many of us, the response would be, "You're crazy. There's no way I can do that!" Now factor in the thought process of an elder who might be confined to a wheelchair or has Parkinson's disease, who uses a walker or a cane, who is unfamiliar and, frankly, uncomfortable with creating art. Both a folk and a medical perspective unveils a deeper understanding of and appreciation for the hesitancy in and the positive power of the art-making process, as well as the material object itself.

Mary Louise Defender Wilson contextualized this traditional dance and MPD project with the story "The Spiderman and the Giant." In brief, Spiderman,

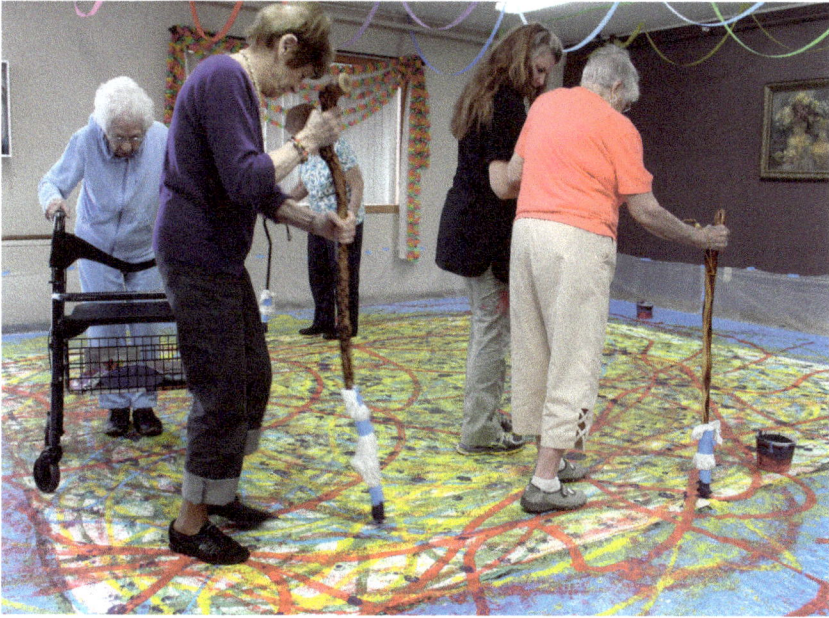

Fig. 10.5. Maureen McDonald-Hins leads elders in a group Irish dance; leaving marks on the canvas with their feet, canes, shillelaghs, and strollers dipped in paint, Enderlin, North Dakota. *Courtesy of North Dakota Council on the Arts.*

a Dakota culture hero, was walking along and found a sleeping, snoring giant. Climbing upon the nose of the giant and peering into his mouth, Spiderman was astonished to find entire villages of people. These people were living their lives unaware that they had been consumed and were now living inside the giant. The giant awoke and told Spiderman that he was hungry and was going to eat another village full of people just over the hill.

During their visit, Spiderman discovered four things the giant was afraid of: the sounds of singing, the drum, the rattle, and the whistle. While the giant continued to rest, Spiderman ran to the next village to warn the people. He advised them to sing and play their instruments when the giant arrived. As the giant approached, the people did as they were instructed, whereupon the giant, surprised and terrified, immediately perished from fright.

In the story, the giant is anything that restricts any one of us from reaching our true potential. Sometimes when people are placed in an eldercare facility, a hospital, a wheelchair, or some other situation, they may perceive those things as large, unwieldy, and scary "giants" that consume and constrain us. And, indeed, in some ways, they may be. However, as Mary Louise points out, "Sometimes we let ourselves live inside the giant," not realizing that we are in fact limiting ourselves. All four things that debilitated the giant and awoke the people to their true capacity to live unencumbered and free—the sounds of singing, the drum, the rattle, and the whistle—are arts (Geist 2017, 32).

It must also be noted that other people, whether family or health professionals, may themselves inadvertently limit and constrain the elders they love and care for. Sometimes this is due to the misconceptions we place on the abilities and potential of elders. In many deeply insightful ways, this traditional Dakota story speaks to a healthy response known to the medical world by another name.

The late Gene Cohen was a renowned pioneer in the field of geriatric psychiatry at the George Washington University Center on Aging, Health & Humanities. Dr. Cohen (2006), in an article titled, "Research on Creativity and Aging: The Positive Impact of the Arts on Health and Illness," identifies various factors that creative expression triggers to promote health.

One factor is the "sense of control mechanism." This is a sense of mastery or competency that people feel when they accomplish something they did not think or expect was possible. When they achieve that something, they feel a sense of pride, confidence, ability, and courage to master another activity or achieve another goal. Studies on aging have shown an association with positive health outcomes when a sense of control or mastery is achieved (Cohen 2006, 9).

A related concept is PNI, the mind's influence through the brain and central nervous system to have a physiological impact on the body and immune system. Dr. Cohen (2006, 9) wrote: "PNI scientists view the positive feelings associated with a sense of control as triggering a response in the brain that sends a signal to the immune system to produce more beneficial immune system cells. In effect, a sense of control triggers a boost in immune-system cells, including T cells and NK cells. T cells are small white blood cells that orchestrate or directly participate in the immune defenses. . . . NK cells refer to "natural killer" cells—large granule-filled lymphocytes that attack tumor cells and infected body cells."

After successfully taking part in the completion of a large painting through traditional dance and the MPD, how would you feel? The process and the large material reminders—the paintings themselves—brought smiles, positive feelings, and a sense of accomplishment. Consider the feelings generated within a woman at the Enderlin care facility when she likened her experience to a life-lesson applicable to other difficulties in her life. She described how she literally painted herself into a corner while using an electric wheelchair and the attached MPD. She philosophized that regardless of what hurdles in life come, one can stop, think, and maneuver around it (Geist 2015a).

Or reflect upon an elder in Wahpeton who was residing in the care facility temporarily as she recuperated from injuries. With other residents seated in chairs and wheelchairs arranged in a circle on the canvas, paint was poured at their feet. James LaRocque, seated among them, played Michif fiddle music and

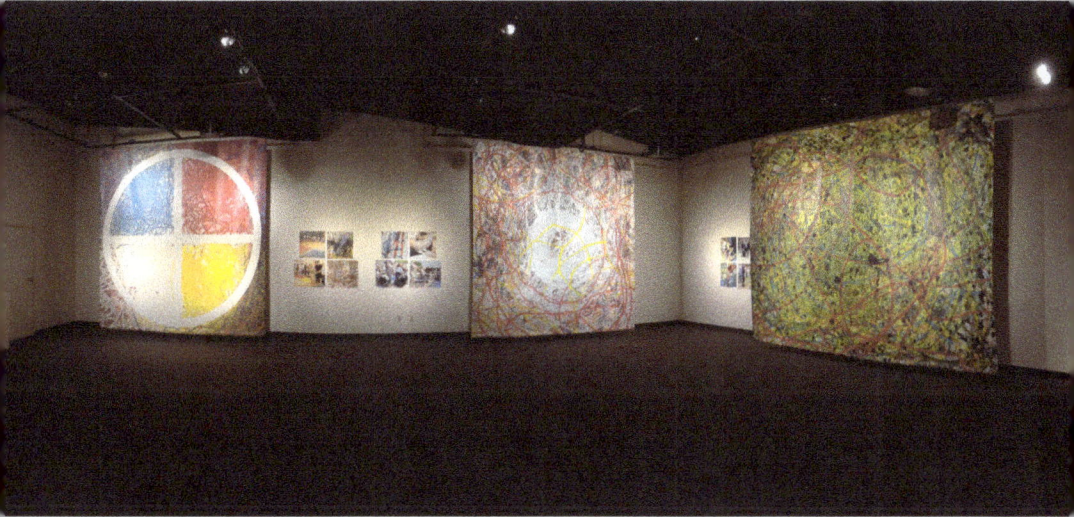

Fig. 10.6. Three of four contemporary paintings, each approximately twelve-by-fifteen feet, on exhibit at the Jamestown Fine Arts Center, Jamestown, North Dakota. *Photograph courtesy of Sally Jeppson.*

demonstrated to the participants how to move their feet to the music in a folk jigging style. Later that night, that same woman was interviewed. With her daughter present, she was asked how she felt and what she thought while participating in the activity.

Smiling broadly, she reminisced about the coolness of the paint squishing through her toes on that hot summer day. And how, as she moved her feet around and looked down upon the paint, she could "see" her children running through mud puddles. Continuing, she stated, "I thought it was so refreshing. Something new I never done in my life. And you're never too old to do something new." Silent for a few seconds and looking into the distance, she explained how she felt: "Just really light. I mean, you had no worries. I don't know. It just made me feel . . . probably like an angel. Gotta be part of heaven" (Geist 2015b).

Working together in the creative process, the seniors clearly accomplished something they did not think was possible. In so doing through art, they freed themselves from the constraints of their respective "giants," whether that be loneliness, feelings of inadequacy, confinement, or pain. Positive feelings, emotions, and thoughts rose to the surface. They felt better, both emotionally and, if PNI is to be considered, physiologically as well, if even for a short time.

After the paintings were completed, the artwork was developed, along with photographs, into an exhibit (fig. 10.6) that toured to each participating community and was featured in local art festivals. Receptions for the senior artists were held. Thus, the objects themselves, the paintings, again served as visual reminders of the elders' accomplishments, which sparked anew those positive feelings and emotions. Thus, both process and object are important for impact. Each painting now resides with the corresponding facility where it was originally created.

The second project example to be highlighted is Tree of Life: Traditional Papercutting, Nostalgia, and Life Review. This Art for Life Program plan and activity was conducted in partnership with the arts council and eldercare facility in Jamestown, North Dakota, in 2016. It was guided by local traditional papercutting artists Meridee Erickson-Stowman and Sabrina Hornung.

Trees are prominent motifs and symbols in traditions, mythologies, and folk cultures around the world. We have all heard the terms *tree of knowledge, tree of life*, and *family tree*. In ancient Norse mythology, there are nine worlds, each connected by the immense, eternally green ash tree Yggdrasil. The lives of humans, gods, and mythic animals play out within these nine realms and all are connected by this "World Tree." In Buddhist mythology, Buddha sat under the Bodhi tree, "the tree of enlightenment," when he received his legendary insight. The Hindu god Vishnu, too, sat under the banyan tree as he taught philosophy and science to humanity. American Indians of the Great Plains receive wisdom as they perform the sun dance around the sacred cottonwood tree. In the Bible's Garden of Eden there grew two trees, the "tree of life" and the "tree of knowledge of good and evil." Today, Christmas and everlasting life is represented by the evergreen tree. All of these examples are illustrative of the tree as a symbol for life's journey, spirituality, and enlightenment.

As such, it is not surprising that the tree of life can be found in traditional songs, music, and arts from around the world. Visually, the designs often depict a tree bursting with life—leaves, flowers, fruit, nuts, birds, and other animals. One of the most colorful and decorative representations of the tree of life can be found in the traditional art of Polish papercutting or wycinanki. This is an art form whereby intricate designs are delicately cut into paper. To hasten the process, the paper is folded in various ways, cut, and then unfolded to reveal complex designs or multiple images. Wycinanki involves the use of many colors of paper layered upon each other in ever-decreasing size to contrast with the material beneath.

The tree of life, both as a metaphor and as a visual motif in folk art, lends itself to use as a vehicle to engage elders in nostalgia and life review, two powerful social-therapeutic modalities. Nostalgia, that wistful longing for the "good old days," often is misunderstood, possibly to the detriment of elders' health. When it was first identified in the late 1600s, it was viewed as a medical malady contributing to anxiety, depression, and irregular heartbeat (Routledge et al. 2011, 298–99). Unfortunately, some such negative sentiments remain today. How often have elders, especially those in care facilities, been perceived as stuck in the past when they repeatedly share their memories? How often have elders been dissuaded from engaging in nostalgic conversations, especially when tears begin to flow? We fear it will initiate depression. We want the elder to be happy, so we steer them away from such topics.

The important work of existential psychologists such as Clay Routledge upends these historic and lingering misconceptions regarding the detrimental impact of nostalgia. Researchers have found that nostalgia, while involving a bit of sadness, actually has a net-positive effect: that nostalgia does not cause negative emotional states but rather is a natural and healthy coping mechanism in response to stressful emotional and physical states. It "elevates positive mood, boosts self-esteem, and strengthens social connectedness" (Routledge et al. 2011, 638). It makes people happier, less lonely, and more optimistic for the future.

In a related vein, life review was developed by the noted gerontologist and psychiatrist Robert N. Butler. It is a developmental process of examining one's life in celebration of its accomplishments and in coping with its disappointments (Haber 2006, 155). It can be facilitated through practices such as storytelling, memoir, autobiography, and nostalgia. Nostalgia affects not only the individual but also the group. As folklorist Ray Cashman (2006, 155) wrote, "Through prolonged and honest engagement with others, however, we come to appreciate the value of the backward glance as an instrument of critical evaluation and of efforts to (re)build community." Individuals who enter care facilities are in stress and often remain separate from others even though they share the same space. Individuals who remain in stress create a community in stress. Initiating shared nostalgic experiences between individuals can bind them together creating a healthier and happier person and, collectively, a healthier and happier community.

Informed by the benefits of nostalgia and life review, residents at the eldercare facility in Jamestown were brought together to share and discuss important parts of their lives. The vehicle for this interaction and reminiscence was the creation of a seven-foot-tall wycinanki tree of life papercutting. The project started with a bare tree trunk and branches made of paper adhered to a canvas with Mod Podge. Every week the elders gathered in small groups around tables. Their discussions and artistic work were led by eldercare and art council staff, volunteers (including children), and the traditional papercutting artists.

Each meeting focused on reminiscing about a specific life event or theme, especially the traditions and beliefs associated with those experiences. Led by the wycinanki artists (fig. 10.7), the elders created papercuttings symbolic of the topic of discussion. The art making facilitated and served as a vehicle for the nostalgic interaction. Conversations ranged from the roots of the elder's family tree (depicted by acorns) to love and marriage (shown by doves and flowers) to starting a family and having children (illustrated by peacocks [fig. 10.8] and red

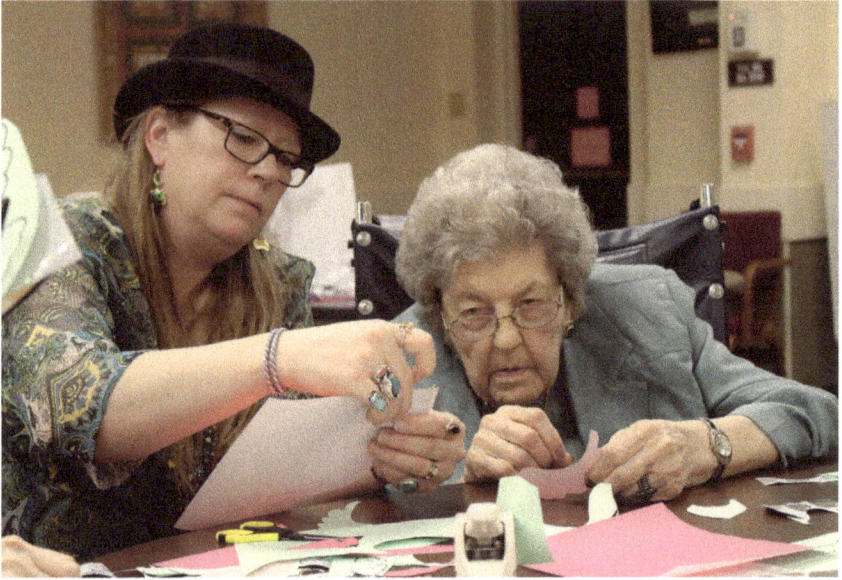

Fig. 10.7. Meridee Erikson Stowman, wycinanki artist, demonstrates papercutting for an elder in a care facility in Jamestown, North Dakota. *Courtesy of North Dakota Council on the Arts.*

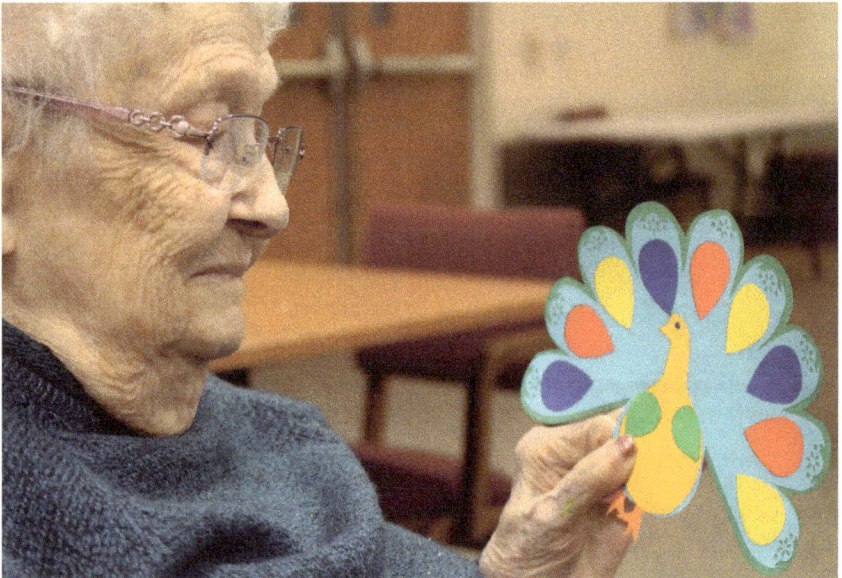

Fig. 10.8. An elder admires her peacock papercutting, Jamestown, North Dakota. *Courtesy of North Dakota Council on the Arts.*

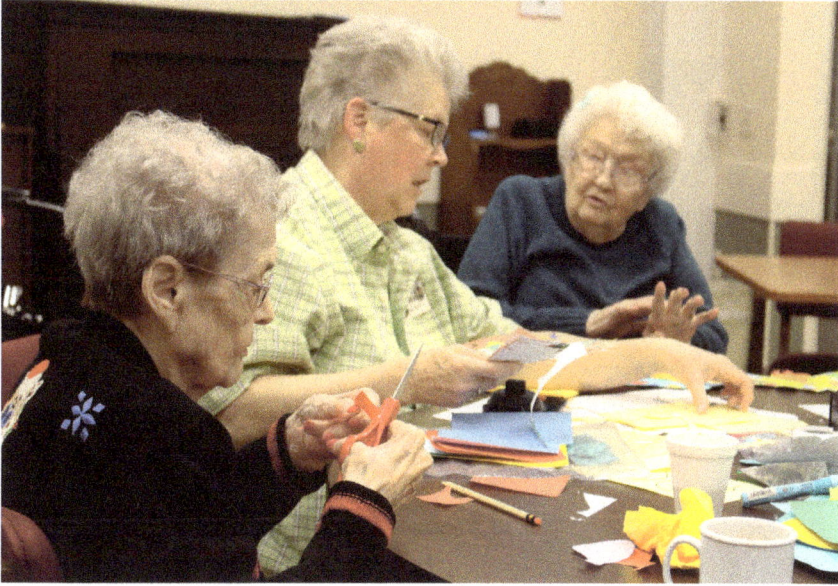

Fig. 10.9. Participation in the Tree of Life project results in frequent discussions bringing elders together over shared experiences, which allows them to forge stronger relationships. *Courtesy of North Dakota Council on the Arts.*

apples) to the end of life and what comes after (insinuated with roosters crowing in a new day).

The conversations all involved folklore and traditions. While visiting about anniversaries, for instance, golden birthdays were shared and papercuttings of golden apples or pears were created. Beliefs about birds crashing into windows as an omen for an impending death, visitations by deceased relatives, or being saved from mishap by a guardian angel were some of the subjects shared during talks about life after death. The session on love and marriage included recollections of shivaree, bidding on the bride's garter, and other wedding traditions.

Multiple senses were utilized to enliven the elders' capacity to remember and willingness to interact with one another (fig. 10.9). Have you ever smelled something and instantly a pleasant memory flashes to mind? This is referred to as odor-evoked autobiographical memory or the Proust phenomenon. Researchers who study this experience state that as olfactory stimuli travel to the brain, they stimulate the brain's emotion and memory centers (Masaoka et al. 2012, 379). Researchers such as Masaoka and colleagues (2012, 387) further state that positive odor-evoked autobiographical memories may be stored in long-term memory, and their recall are associated with slow and deep breathing beneficial for feeling relaxed in stressful situations.

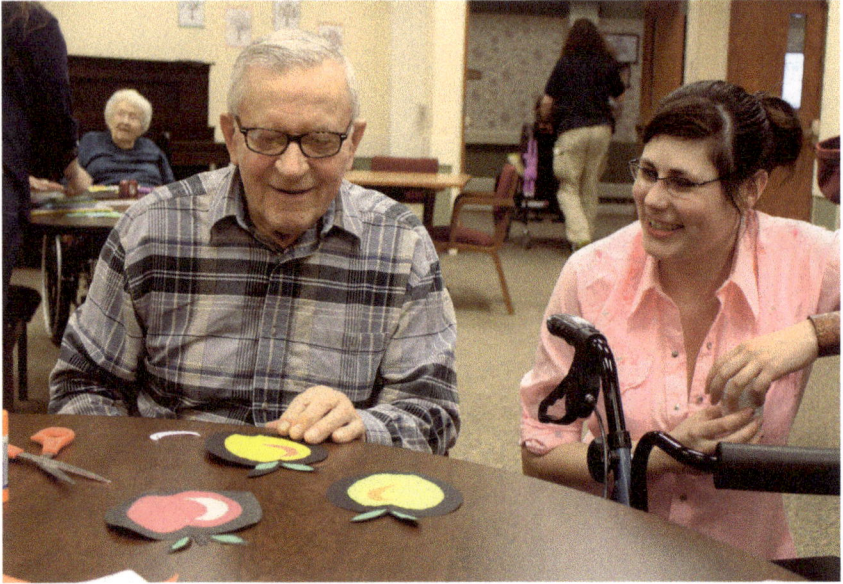

Fig. 10.10. An elder in a care facility in Jamestown, North Dakota, completes three of four apple papercuttings—one for each of his children—as wycinanki artist Sabrina Hornung looks on. *Courtesy of North Dakota Council on the Arts.*

When love and marriage was discussed and papercuttings of doves were made, a wedding cake was baked and served to those in attendance. When having children was the topic and papercuttings of apples were made (fig. 10.10), warm fragrant apple turnovers were served. The cake and turnovers functioned not only as a polite social courtesy, as food often brings people together in a harmonious way, but as a focused effort to enliven both the memory and body through sight, taste, and smell. This contributed to both the success of the process and the completion of the art piece.

At the end of each session, that day's thematic artwork was added to the paper tree on the canvas. As each gathering passed, the traditional artists arranged the artwork so that the tree grew and blossomed to life (fig. 10.11). Like the traditional dance and painting project described earlier, working together the elders created something very complex and grand in scale that no one person could accomplish alone. Thus, Gene Cohen's sense of control mechanism is again called to mind. Additionally triggered are the positive feelings connected to nostalgia, life review, and the Proust phenomenon. These, in turn, can all be said to be influencers in the positive health benefits associated with PNI.

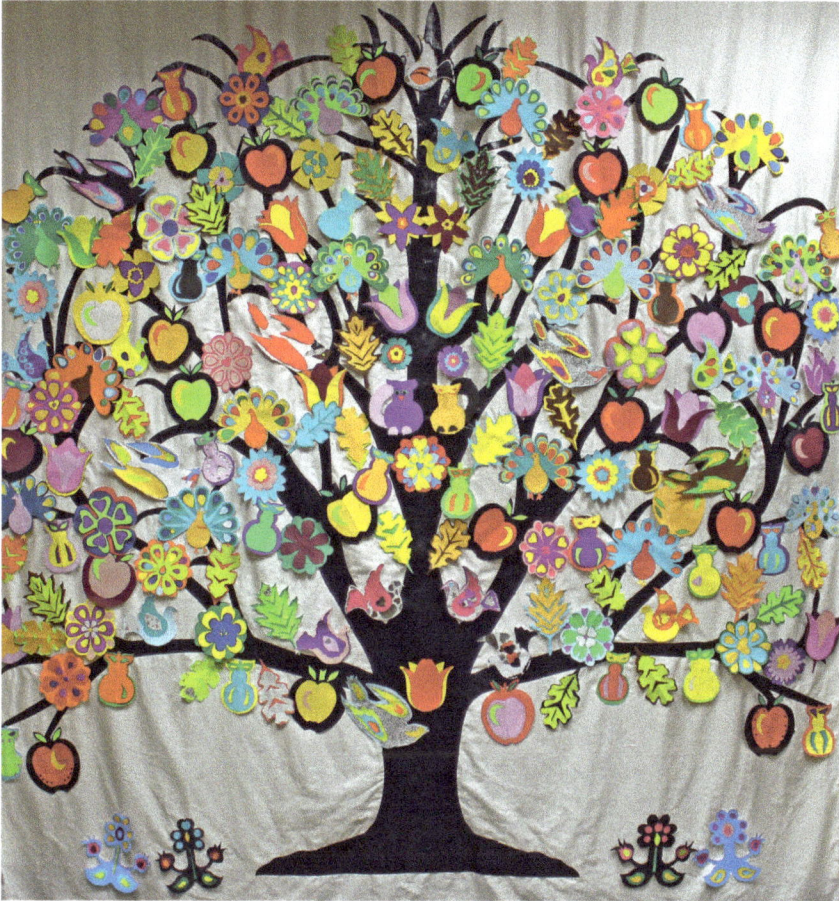

Fig. 10.11. Nearly complete seven-foot-tall Tree of Life papercutting. *Courtesy of North Dakota Council on the Arts.*

In addition, traditions and folk art are powerful vehicles for creative engagement also because they hold a place in already existing, ongoing social relationships and structures. Let us make a comparison to brain plasticity—the ability
of the brain to adapt by forming and strengthening new cells and connection
points. Gene Cohen (2006, 10) wrote:

> When the brain is challenged through our activities and surroundings, it is
> altered through the formation of new synapses (contact points between cells).
> More synapses means better communication among brain cells and increased

**Pathways and Points of Interaction**

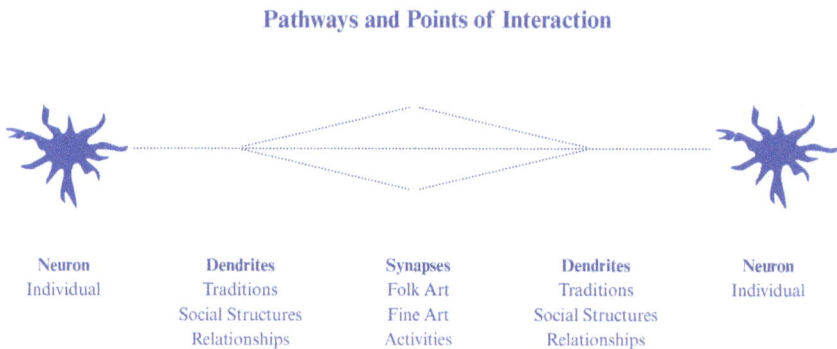

| Neuron | Dendrites | Synapses | Dendrites | Neuron |
|---|---|---|---|---|
| Individual | Traditions | Folk Art | Traditions | Individual |
| | Social Structures | Fine Art | Social Structures | |
| | Relationships | Activities | Relationships | |

Fig. 10.12. *Courtesy of North Dakota Council on the Arts.*

opportunities for new ideas connecting. When branchlike extensions (known as dendrites) from one brain cell (neuron) achieve contact with extensions of other neurons, new synapses are formed. Challenging activities and new experiences induce the sprouting of new dendrites, thereby enhancing brain reserve. Art activities are especially good because they are more likely to be sustained, and just like the impact of physical exercise over the long term, the benefits of challenges for the brain increase when they are ongoing.

Within the context of the tree of life project:

Now think of neurons as individuals or elders and dendrites as social relationships facilitated through social structures embedded in traditions, these being pathways for interaction and communication that connect neurons to one another. Think of folk arts as synapses that serve as contact points between cells, or between individuals [fig. 10.12]. The more contact points, the better the communication and social engagement. Because social relationships, social structures, and activities associated with traditions such as holidays and folk arts already exist, they are more likely to be sustained in meaningful ways over the life cycle to the benefit of the elder. The stronger and healthier the pathways for communication and interaction, the better the elders can adapt to challenges, i.e. 'brain reserve.' For elders to live on their own or in care facilities, these structures and relationships, both old and new, must be supported and formed. They can be strengthened and created through traditions, folk art, and fine art. (Geist 2017, 40)

Once again, and in conclusion, when working with material folk art and elders, (1) the creative process as well as the final object itself are crucial to impact; (2) activating the five senses, sometimes by integrating nonmaterial folk arts, folklore, or traditions such as food, music, or dance, can help enliven the elder in the process and toward the completion of the material art; and (3) interaction between elders in care facilities must be fostered. The creation of folk art with these points in mind can contribute uniquely to the health and wellness of elders—decreasing loneliness, strengthening social connectedness, elevating positive mood, combatting stress, triggering memories, boosting the immune system, and much more.

Folk traditions and folk arts have a power all their own. Our emotional and physiological responses to art interventions that involve nostalgia or positive odor-evoked autobiographical memories and the resulting effects of PNI, for instance, are in many ways culturally determined. The taste and smell of certain traditional foods may be deemed pleasant by some while unpleasant by others. Music associated with one's culture growing up has a personal connection to an elder growing older, enlivening them psychologically and physiologically. The fond nostalgic memories of childhood and young adulthood often cluster around holidays, cultural customs, and family traditions. Knowledge of an elder's traditional background and the traditions of various peoples can facilitate nostalgia, spark memories, and bring lonely people together. Thus, folklorists who are knowledgeable and trained in understanding the complexities of traditions, folk arts, and cultural context within the lives of people hold an important, perhaps critical, place in the world of potent creative aging and health programming.

TROYD GEIST is State Folklorist at the North Dakota Council on the Arts. He originated and developed the Art for Life Program and is the coauthor of *Sundogs and Sunflowers: Folklore and Folk Art of the Northern Great Plains*.

## Works Cited

Cashman, Ray. 2006. "Critical Nostalgia and Material Culture in Northern Ireland." *The Journal of American Folklore* 119 (472): 137–60.

Cohen, Gene D. 2006. "Research on Creativity and Aging: The Positive Impact of the Arts on Health and Illness." *Generations: Journal of the American Society on Aging* 30 (1): 7–15.

Geist, Troyd A. 2015a. *Yes, I Am Free: The Inspiration of Dance and Paint* (project video interview of participants). Enderlin: North Dakota Council on the Arts, June 6.

Geist, Troy A. 2015b. *Yes, I Am Free: The Inspiration of Dance and Paint* (project video interview of participants). Wahpeton: North Dakota Council on the Arts, June 8. https://vimeopro.com/user14965043/north-dakota-council-on-the-arts/video /138253051.

Geist, Troyd A. 2017. *Sundogs and Sunflowers: An Art for Life Program Guide for Creative Aging, Health, and Wellness*. Bismarck: North Dakota Council on the Arts.

Haber, David. 2006. "Life Review: Implementation, Theory, Research, and Therapy." *International Journal of Aging and Human Development* 63 (2): 153–71.

Masaoka, Y., H. Sugiyama, A. Katayama, M. Kashiwagi, and I. Homma. 2012. "Slow Breathing and Emotions Associated with Odor-Induced Autobiographical Memories." *Chemical Senses* 37 (4): 379–88.

Routledge, Clay, Jamie Arndt, Tim Wildschut, Constantine Sedikides, Claire M. Hart, Jacob Juhl, Ad. J. J. M. Vingerhoets, and Wolff Schlotz. 2011. "The Past Makes the Present Meaningful: Nostalgia as an Existential Resource." *Journal of Personality and Social Psychology* 101 (3): 638–52.

Thomas, William. 1999. *The Eden Alternative Handbook: The Art of Building Human Habitats*. Sherburne, NY: Summer Hill.

# Index

Abram, David, 164
American Folklore Society, ix, 9–10
andragogy, 182
applied folklore, 11–14, 24n5. *See also* public
    folklore
apprenticeships, 12–13, 28, 33, 35, 38, 81, 84,
    87, 91, 93, 100, 103–104, 179, 187–188
Arriola, Martha, 125–126
Arroyo Lugo José, 55–71, 74–78
Art for Life Program, 12, 90, 189, 196

Bailey, David, 165–168
Baker, Lillie Liston, 115–116
Baltes, Paul and Margaret, 16
Bateman, Mary Josephine Wilson, 116
Bauman, Richard, 3
Ben-Amos, Dan, 3
Bentz, Joann, 145–146
Bloomquist, Pieper, 188
boredom, 2, 28, 104, 143, 149–150, 188
Bossenberger, Eva, 146
*botánica*, 46–48, 51, 54n5
Brady, Leah, 86
Bronner, Simon, 11, 19
Bryan, Cliff, 28
Bryant, Marie, 146
Bustin, Dillon, 11
Butler, Robert, 12, 182, 197
Byrd, Cindy, 154

Cashman, Ray, 197
Chaney, Arlene Flynn, 107–108, 114, 136n5
Cobb, Edith, 169
Coggswell, Gladys, 29
Cohen, Gene, 4–5, 27–28, 97, 177–178, 194,
    200–201
Collins, Mary Alice, 18–19
Cote, Tom, 180–182
Cowen, Olen, 5
Creative Aging Network, 27
cultural disruption, 88, 90

Dala painting, 188
Dégh, Linda, 5
Dence, Sofia, 29
Dickie, Virginia, 142–143
Dobson, Liza, 109, 111, 114, 129, 136n3, 136n7
Donaldson, Beth, 143
Douglas, Gladys Gorman, 8–9
Drevs, Everett, 144–145
Duncan, Fumiko, 84, 88–89
Duntan, WIlliam R, 142

Eaton, Allen, 19–20
Erickson, Erik, 7, 13, 176, 178, 182
*Espiritismo*, 43, 53n1
Evans, Mary Louis, 122–124

Festival of American Folklife. *See* Smithso-
    nian Folklife Festival
folk arts, 20, 28, 56, 74–75, 88, 153–154, 178,
    186–187, 189, 202–203
foodways, 16, 44–45, 86, 88, 189; food pres-
    ervation, 106–137; food-based reciprocity,
    114–117
Frazier, Doris, 29

gardening, 106–137
Geist, Troyd, 12, 27–28, 90–91, 178
generativity, 7–9, 179–180
gerontology, 4, 11, 13–14, 90, 141, 153; folklor-
    istic, 9, 13–16
Glassie, Henry, 5
Goldstein, Kenneth, 13
Graber, LeRoy, 5
Graves, Don, 29

Hall, Glenn, 2–3
Halperin, Rhoda, 107
Hatton, Clay, 117
Hatton, Hershel Clay, 107
Havighurst, Robert, 12
Hawes, Bess Lomax, 10

helplessness, 2, 149, 188
Helton, Damon, 6–7
heritage, 70–71, 178–179
Herring, Charles, 84
Higgins, Rita Rae, 111–112
Honeycutt, James Espen, 5
Hufford, Barbara, 154–155
Hufford, David, 12–13
Hufford, Mary, 10, 12, 108, 176, 178
Hughes, Trudie, 146
Hunley, Robert, 6
Hunt, Marjorie, 10, 12, 153, 176, 178

Ike, Roger, 86
isolation. *See* loneliness

Jabbour, Alan, 5, 11, 137n19, 178
Jones, Alfred, 111
Jones, Michael Owen, 89–90

Kane, Richard, 11
Kay, Jon, 27–28, 66, 74, 77n6, 90, 105n3, 178
Kentucky Folklife Program, 5, 7
Kimball, Hattie, 116
Kirshenblatt-Gimblett, Barbara, 9, 12, 154, 178
Knowles, Malcolm, 181–182

Lassila, Anna, 95–105
Ledbetter, Huddie "Ledbelly," 5
life review, 182–183, 189, 196–197, 200
Lomax, Alan, 5
loneliness, 4, 51, 149, 188, 195, 197, 203
Lynn, Joyce, 145–146

material legacies, 37
Mathers Museum of World Cultures, 15
memory objects, 35, 58–61, 78n15
Michigan State University Museum's Traditional Arts Program, 100, 103
Miller, Ellis Cool, 108–109
Miller, Howard, 129
Miller, Sadie, 113–114
Miracle, James, 5
Missouri, 27, 30–32, 35, 38
Missouri Traditional Arts Apprenticeship program, 35, 38, 40
Mohamed, Ethel, 10, 154
Morales, Jerusalén, 42–54

Morgan, Nancy, 18–19
Moses, Grandma, 4–5
Mullen, Patrick, 11
Muncy, Mossy, 5
Mundell, Kathleen, 12–13
Myerhoff, Barbara, 6, 8, 10, 153

Nachtigall, Jeff, 189–190
Neuhouser, Ruth, 17, 19
Nolan, Hugh, 5
North Dakota Arts Council, 12
North Dakota Council on the Arts (NDCA), 186–187
nostalgia, 196–197

O'Neill, John, 168, 170
Oring, Elliot, 90

Paiute, 80, 86–87, 91–93
Palko, Zsuzsanna, 5
Parker, Molly Neptune, 175, 179–180
Passamaquoddy tribe, 175, 179–180
Patrickus, Joseph Jr., 30–40
Penobscot, 179
Pierce, Elijah, 10
Plagues (of aging), 2, 188
Preston, Ella, 124, 126
psychology, 16
public folklore, 3, 10–11, 40, 153
Puerto Rico, 43

quality of life, 2, 11–13

Reed, Henry, 5
Robbins, Christa, 28–29
Roberts, Katherine, 109
Routledge, Clay, 197
Rural Folklife Days, 1–2, 7–8

Sanders, Virginia, 27
Scharfenberg, Leona, 140
Schoolman, John, 5
Severt, Carrie, 114
Shoshone, 86
Shuldiner, David, 11
Simmons, Philip, 4
Sisters of the Cloth, 8–9
Smithsonian Folklife Festival, 2, 8–10, 97–100

Stephen Foster Folk Culture Center, 1
Synapse Program, 142

Taylor, Bob, 4–5, 15
Tibbs, Sid, 6
Tobey, Hilman, 80, 91–93, 94n1
Traditional Arts Indiana, 18, 74

University of Illinois, Urbana-
    Champaign, 65
University of Puerto Rico (UPR), 64–65

Variakojis, Vilius, 10

Veintidós, Delia Esther Lorenzo, 62, 64–66,
    70–71

Wanner, Hilda, 146
Wells, Hattie, 124
White, Ruth, 148–149, 152n2
Williams, Mike, 88
Wilson, Mary Louise Defender, 192–193
wycinanki, 196–197

Yang, James Min-Ching, 15

Zeitlin, Steven, 10, 12, 153, 176, 178
Zetaruk, Zoria, 86

www.ingramcontent.com/pod-product-compliance
Lightning Source LLC
Chambersburg PA
CBHW040254290326
41929CB00051B/3379